Optavia Diet Cookbook

The Complete 30-Day Rapid Weight Loss Program Challenge to Burn Stubborn Belly Fat, Kill Binge Eating Disorder and Kickstart Your Lifelong Body Transformation. Effortless Lean & Green Recipes On a Budget

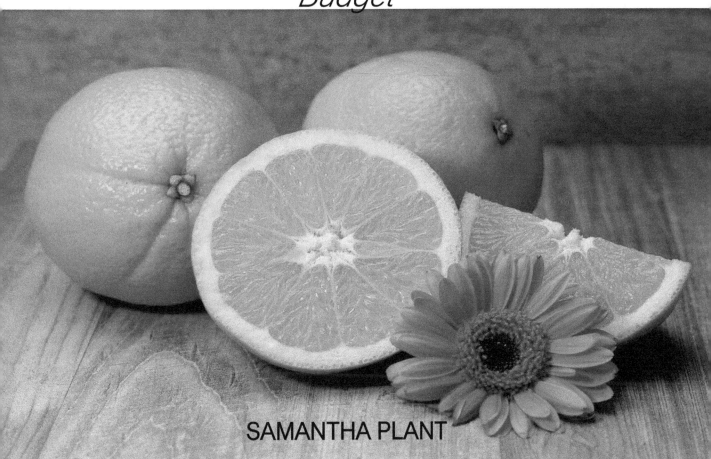

SAMANTHA PLANT

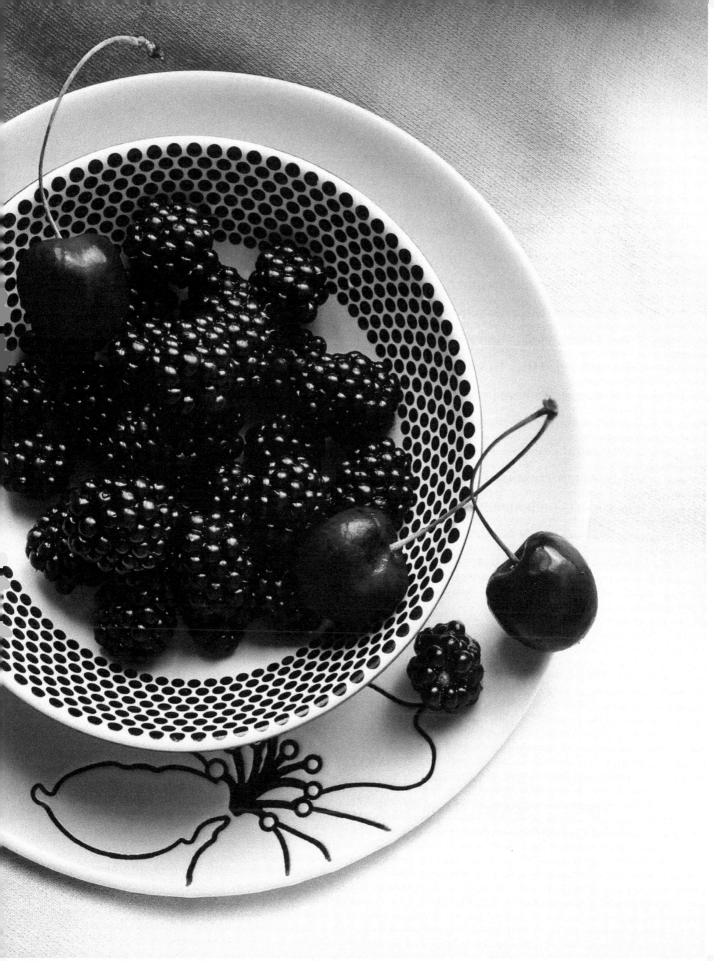

Table of Content

Introduction 1

Chapter 1: How Does The Optavia Diet Work? 2

Chapter 2: Benefits of the Optavia Diet 3

    1. Packaged products offer convenience 3

    2. Achieve rapid weight loss 3

    3. Eliminate the guesswork 3

    4. Offers social support 3

Chapter 3: How to succeed with the Optavia Diet 4

    Measuring Intensity 6

    How many exercises Do You Need to Be Doing? 6

    General Exercise Tips 6

    Strength Training Tips 8

    The 10 Components of Fitness 10

    Benefits of Exercise 13

Chapter 4: Food list – What is allowed and what is not 16

    Lean Meals.. 17

    Green Meal 17

    Foods/Nourishment to keep away from...18

Chapter 5: Which is the Perfect Plan for You? 19

    The 5-and-1 Plan...19

    The 4-and-2-and-1 Plan 20

    The 3-and-3 Plan 21

Chapter 6: The 30-Day Rapid Weight Loss Program Challenge 23

Chapter 7: Breakfast Recipes.. 26

    Breakfast One - Breakfast Hash...26

    Breakfast Two - Breakfast Cookies 26

Breakfast Three - Protein Shake: Vanilla Cashew 27

Breakfast Four - Zucchini Pancakes 28

Breakfast Five - High Protein Pudding 29

Breakfast Six - Breakfast Tacos 30

Breakfast Seven - Blueberry Muffins 31

Breakfast Eight - Green Smoothie 32

Breakfast Nine - Bread Recipe, One 32

Breakfast Ten - Eggs and Toast 33

Breakfast Eleven - Chickpea Skillet 34

Breakfast Twelve - Chocolate Overnight Oats 35

Breakfast Thirteen - Protein Smoothie Bowl 36

Breakfast Fourteen - Peanut Butter Toast 36

Breakfast Fifteen- Light Breakfast, Zero Prep 37

Breakfast Sixteen - Protein Pancakes 38

Breakfast Seventeen - Egg Muffins 38

Breakfast Eighteen - Granola Cereal 39

Breakfast Nineteen - Strawberry Banana Smoothie 40

Breakfast Twenty - Lemon Doughnuts 41

Breakfast Twenty-One- Cream Cheese Recipe 42

Breakfast Twenty-Two- Breakfast Sweet Potatoes 43

Breakfast Twenty-Three- Chia Pudding 43

Breakfast Twenty-Four- Cheesy Casserole 44

Breakfast Twenty-Five - French Toast 45

Breakfast Twenty-Six - Overnight Oats 46

Breakfast Twenty-Seven - Scrambled Tofu 47

Breakfast Twenty-Eight Quinoa & Chocolate Breakfast Bowl 49

Breakfast Twenty-Nine Quinoa & Cinnamon Breakfast Bowl 50

Breakfast Thirty - Fluffy Vegan Pancakes 52

Chapter 8: Lunch Recipes 54

Lunch One - Caesar Salad 54

Lunch Two - Buffalo Chickpeas...55

Lunch Three - Veg Wrap 56

Lunch Four- Egg Salad 56

Lunch Five- Lunch Tacos 57

Lunch Six - Protein Bowl 58

Lunch Seven - Pesto Panini 58

Lunch Eight - Pasta Salad 59

Lunch Nine - Stuffed Sweet Potatoes... 60

Lunch Ten - Stir Fry 61

Lunch Eleven - Chicken Salad...62

Lunch Twelve - Mushroom Soup 63

Lunch Thirteen - Nachos 63

Lunch Fourteen - Lunchbox 64

Lunch Fifteen - Sushi Spring Rolls 65

Lunch Sixteen - Barbeque Chickpea Salad with Ranch 66

Lunch Seventeen - Meatball Bomber 67

Lunch Eighteen - Tomato Soup 68

Lunch Nineteen - Caprese Mozzarella Recipe 69

Lunch Twenty - Avocado Toast 70

Lunch Twenty-One - Taco Meat 71

Lunch Twenty-Two - Creamy Cauliflower Soup.................................. 71

Lunch Twenty-Three - Power Bowl 72

Lunch Twenty-Four - Mediterranean Sandwich 73

Lunch Twenty-Five - Curry 74

Lunch Twenty-Six - Crispy Tofu 75

Lunch Twenty-Seven Thai Noodle Salad 76

Lunch Twenty-Eight - Black Bean Taco Salad.....................................78

Lunch Twenty-Nine - Curried Tofu Salad 80

Lunch Thirty Middle Eastern Chickpea Salad 81

Lunch Thirty-One - Crunchy Veggie Wrap with Apples and Spicy Hummus 82

Lunch Thirty-Two - VBLT—Vegan-Bacon Lettuce and Tomato Sandwich 83

Lunch Thirty-Three - Chickpea Noodle Soup 84

Lunch Thirty-Four - Mexican Lentil Soup 85

Chapter 9: Dinner Recipes **87**

Dinner One - Broccoli Cheese Dish 87

Dinner Two - Mushroom Stew..88

Dinner Three - Baked Ziti 89

Dinner Four - Vegan Chili 90

Dinner Five - Alfredo Sauce Recipe 91

Dinner Six - Fajitas...92

Dinner Seven - Meatless Meatloaf 93

Dinner Eight - Veggie Burger...94

Dinner Nine - Tuna Salad 95

Dinner Ten - Instant Pot Pasta 95

Dinner Eleven - Peanut Tofu with Rice 96

Dinner Twelve - Spicy Tahini Pasta...97

Dinner Thirteen - Sushi Bowl 98

Dinner Fourteen - Lasagna Rollups 100

Dinner Fifteen - Stroganoff..101

Dinner Sixteen - Eggplant Curry 102

Dinner Seventeen - Pizza Crust Recipe 103

Dinner Eighteen - Creamy Potato Soup 103

Dinner Nineteen - Mac n' Cheese 104

Dinner Twenty - Sesame Chickpeas 105

Dinner Twenty-One - Buffalo Bites 106

Dinner Twenty-Two - Black Bean Soup 107

Dinner Twenty-Three - Lentil Bolognese...108

Dinner Twenty-Four - Instant Pot Wild Rice Soup...................................109

Dinner Twenty-Five - Fried Rice...110

Dinner Twenty-Six - Seitan...111

Dinner Twenty-Seven - Buddha Bowl With Peanut Tofu...........................113

Dinner Twenty-Eight - Party Friendly Vegan Pho..................................115

Dinner Twenty-Nine - Vegan Pizza..116

Dinner Thirty - Creamy Garlic and Lemon Fettuccine Alfredo...................118

Dinner Thirty-One - Southwest Stuffed Peppers...................................119

Chapter 10: Snacks & Dessert Recipes..............................**121**

Snack 1 - Spinach and Artichoke Dip...121

Snack Two - Buffalo Dip..122

Snack Three - Potato Wedges..123

Snack Four - Dill Hummus..123

Snack Five - Latte Pudding..124

Snack Six - Peanut Butter...125

Snack Seven - Vegan Crackers...126

Dessert One - Blondies..127

Dessert Two - Peanut Butter Cups..128

Dessert Three - Chocolate Mug Cake..129

Dessert Four - Ice Cream..129

Dessert Five - Chocolate Chip Cookies...130

Dessert Six - Vanilla Cupcakes...131

Dessert Seven - Edible Cookie Dough...132

Dessert Eight - Fat Bomb..133

Dessert Nine - Fruit and Yogurt Parfait...134

Peanut Butter and Chocolate Fudge...135

Dessert Ten - Vegan Apple Crisp..135

Dessert Eleven - Healthy Oatmeal Cookies..137

Dessert Twelve - No-Bake Chocolate Vegan Brownies..................................138

Chapter 11: Recipes for Before & After Workouts **141**

  Preworkout Recipes.. **141**

    Preworkout: One - Peanut Butter Toast 141

    Preworkout: Two - Tropical Smoothie 141

    Preworkout: Three - Apple Slices and Almond Butter............................ 142

    Preworkout: Four - Peanut Butter Toast 143

    Preworkout: Five - Orange and Nuts... 143

  Postworkout Recipes **144**

    Postworkout: One - BodyBuilding Smoothie 144

    Postworkout: Two - Spinach Salad with Tempeh 144

    Postworkout: Three - Steel Cut Oats 145

    Postworkout: Four - Protein Bar 146

    Postworkout: Five - Hummus and Veggies 147

Conclusion **148**

Conversion Charts **149**

Introduction

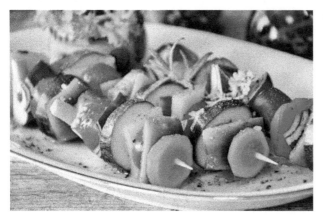

The Optavia diet is a practice aimed at either reducing or maintaining one's current weight. It recommends eating processed food referred to as "Fuelings" and homemade meals "lean and green meal" for dinner. It is believed that sticking to the brand's product "Fuelings" and supplementing a meal with meat, veggies, and a fat entrée every day it will keep you full and adequately nourished. There are no worries about losing muscles as you'll be eating a lot of protein and consuming few calories, about 800 to 1,000 for adults.

With this plan the individuals involved can lose about 12 pounds in just 12 weeks using the 5 & 1 optimal weight plan.

Put simply, the Optavia diet is a program that focuses on lowering calories and the reduction of carbohydrates. Doing this effectively combines packed food called "Fuelings" with homemade meals, thus encouraging loss of weight. The name Optavia sounds like a new drug or an eye-wear brand however it is a weight loss program that has become famous thanks to the internet. Google named Optavia one of the hottest diets of 2018 in its year-end report and Cake Boss Star Buddy Valastro said he lost weight thanks to this program.

Optavia adds a social support component with access to a health coach who can answer questions and give encouragement.

In addition, the plan also recommends doing about 30 minutes of moderate intensity exercise a day.

The company claims that by working with its coaches and following a diet that includes OPTAVIA products, "a permanent transformation" is achieved.

Chapter 1: How Does The Optavia Diet Work?

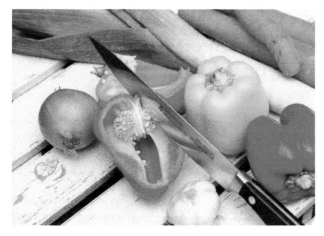

Most people follow the 5 & 1 program that incorporates five refills per day. With this program, customers eat 5 of Optavia's "supplies" and one lean and green low- calorie homemade meal per day.

You can also choose more than 60 options, including smoothies, bars, soups, cookies, and pudding, including high-quality protein and one probiotic that the brand claims to aid digestive health. Your sixth daily meal (that you can eat at any time) is built around cooked lean protein, three servings of non-starchy vegetables, and healthy fats.

During the diet, you will work with Optavia trainers and join a community to share your success. Once you've reached your weight goal, transitioning from the plan should be more comfortable as healthier ones replace your old habits. Optavia offers a specific product line through its 3 and 3 plans for weight maintenance.

For people who want a more flexible and high-calorie diet, OPTAVIA suggests the 4 & 2 & 1 plan that incorporates four meals, two lean and green meals, and one healthy snack, like a baked potato or fruit.

Optavia also sells specific programs for people with diabetes, nursing moms, the elderly and teenagers.

Chapter 2: Benefits of the Optavia Diet

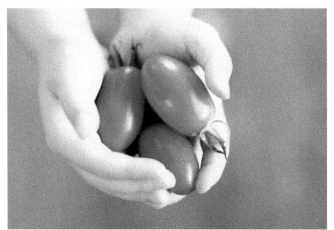

1. Packaged products offer convenience

Optavia's smoothies, soups, and other meal replacement products are shipped to your door providing a level of convenience that many other diets don't offer.

Even if you will need to purchase your Ingredients for "lean and green" meals, Optavia's home delivery option for "supplies" helps a lot.

Once the products arrive, they are easy to prepare and make great takeaway meals.

2. Achieve rapid weight loss

Most healthy people need around 1,600-3,000 calories per day to maintain their weight. Limiting that amount to a minimum of 800 guarantees weight loss for most people.

Optavia's 5 & 1 plan is designed for rapid weight loss, making it a viable option for someone with a medical reason to lose weight fast.

3. Eliminate the guesswork

Some people say that the most challenging part of a diet is the mental effort to figure out what to eat each day or at each meal.

Optavia relieves the stress of meal planning and "decision fatigue" by offering users approved foods with "supplies" and guidelines for "lean and green" meals.

4. Offers social support

Social support is an essential component of the success of any weight loss program. Optavia's coaching program and group call ensure integrated encouragement and support for users.

Chapter 3: How to succeed with the Optavia Diet

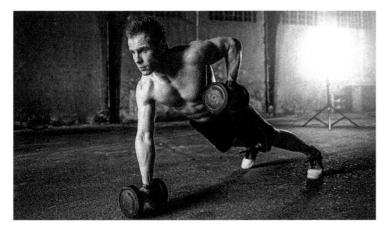

With the Optavia Diet, it is believed you can live the best possible healthy life but requires an effort to keep and maintain a healthy lifestyle.

Optavia diet plan will help you achieve lifelong transformation by incorporating healthy habits into everything you do—these habits get your mind and body working together for you. Every simple new habit, every healthy decision all leads to positive change.

When it is necessary to maintain a healthy lifestyle by losing weight, exercise is essential. During weight loss, you need to burn more calories than you consume. Regular exercise can be so beneficial even to the brain.

You don't have to exercise to lose weight, but it helps. If you decide to add in exercise, you should do a combination of cardio and strength training. Cardio helps you burn more calories and strength training will maintain your muscle. It's essential to preserve muscle as you lose weight because muscle burns calories. If you don't do any strength training, then you'll likely lose muscle as you lose weight.

When you picture someone fit and healthy, what do they look like? Usually, your mind might gravitate towards the image of a person who is chiselled and physically lean. Of course, that person didn't get that way just because they eat salads all day. Yes, dieting is an essential aspect of fitness. There's no doubt about it. However, it's only half the story. Not all of the work that you do towards fitness is done in the kitchen. You also need to be putting in the work at the gym as well.

You need to engage in proper and consistent exercise if you truly want to lose weight.

Sure, in theory, you would be able to lose weight by just dieting alone. However, by merely limiting yourself to dieting and no exercise, you are handicapping your progress. You have an opportunity to accelerate your progress in your weight loss journey if you can combine a strict diet with an effective exercise routine. So, even if you aren't the most athletic person in the world you are going to want to consider the idea of adopting an exercise routine for yourself.

It is going to be challenging to sustain a physically active lifestyle. However, you know that this is something that you need to do for your good. It's incredibly troubling these days in the age of technology that machines are starting to make peoples' lives easier. Yes, there is irony in that sentence. Technology has indeed made the lives of people all around the world so much easier and more convenient. However, it has also encouraged laziness and inactivity among so many people. Why would you do something yourself when a machine can do it on your behalf? Even simple household tasks like sweeping or vacuuming can be done by a robot now. There is just so much more incentive for people to sit still and relax all of the time. This is why so many people end up becoming obese or overweight. They aren't moving enough for them to burn the calories that they need to create a deficit.

This is precisely why the fitness industry is more critical than ever. Since machines are practicing most of the work that human beings used to be responsible for, people now need an outlet to stay physically active. So, to set you on your path to becoming physically fit let's first discuss what constitutes proper training and exercise.

It can get uncomfortable when you're just lugging around a lot of excess weight all of the time. But it's not just the discomfort that you need to worry about. You also need to be taking a good look at your health.

If you're unaware, being obese or overweight can lead to several dangerous diseases such as diabetes, hypertension, kidney disease, cardiovascular disease, stroke, and even cancer. And unfortunately, there are so many people in the world who are overweight these days.

This level of inactivity for the modern human being can be very harmful to one's health. This is why there is a need for people to engage in a strict and effective exercise routine. To make up for the level of inactivity undertaken throughout the rest of the day one must dedicate a few minutes or hours to just engaging in rigorous physical activity. So, this leads to ask the question, what constitutes exercise?

Remember that regular physical activity is different from exercise. The physical activity you engage in every day, like walking to your car or standing up from your desk, is not a form of exercise. Yes, you are exerting a certain amount of effort by recruiting your muscles. But it isn't necessarily vigorous physical activity. Exercise is a physical activity that is more strenuous, planned, and purposeful. However, exercise can mean different things to many different people considering that we all have varying fitness levels. To an overweight older adult walking for 20 minutes might constitute exercise however for a relatively healthy 20-year-old walking for 20 minutes is essentially just regular physical activity. Essentially, it all boils down to the level of intensity that a person is exhibiting while performing any given movement.

Measuring Intensity

You don't have to engage in complex and meticulous quantitative measurements of your physical activity for you to figure out if you're exercising or not. You just merely have to pay attention to how you are feeling. To simplify things, you can classify intensity into two different categories: moderate and vigorous. If you perform a movement and are having difficulty breathing, but can still talk while doing it, then it's moderate intensity. However, when you try hard to catch your breath to the point that you can't talk anymore, you are engaged in vigorous intensity. When engaging in active exercise, you should aim to be giving an emotional level of intensity.

How many exercises Do You Need to Be Doing?

For you to be able to reap the benefits of engaging in exercise, you need to develop a routine for yourself. This routine should have you performing some kind of aerobic or anaerobic exercise at least three times a week. For each of these sessions, you should try to make them last for as long as 30 minutes to an hour. The more intense and the longer your workout the more calories you will burn actively. Hence, with the additional calories than you are burning the faster you will lose weight.

General Exercise Tips

1. Find a Routine You Enjoy

You're not going to work out consistently if you hate doing it. So, explore different apps, machines, and routines until you find a few that you like. It's OK to stick to those for a while until they get easy or boring. Then you can switch it up with something new.

2. Keep Your Goal in Mind

When you're feeling too lazy to exercise, it's easy to forget why you're even doing it in the first place. Instead of just forcing yourself to work out, try to visualize how your body will look and how you'll feel from all your effort.

3. Start Slow

If you lack the motivation to work out, then don't agonize about it. Set small goals for yourself just to get in the habit or tell yourself that it's just this one time for a few minutes. Once you start the workout, you'll feel good from the endorphins that it triggers. You'll want to keep up the habit.

4. Set Up Triggers

Your reward censer will remember the feeling it gets from a workout. You can trigger the craving for that feeling by leaving out your gym clothes or workout equipment. You're more likely to exercise if you make the process as convenient as possible.

5. Hydrate

Make sure you're hydrated before the workout and have water on you at all times. Dehydration will cause you to burn out too quickly.

6. Stretch

Stretch after your workouts so that you're not too sore from exercising the next day. Hold each stretch for 20-30 seconds. Start the stretch gently, at a point where it doesn't cause discomfort. Then gradually stretch the muscle even further every few seconds as it loosens.

7. Re-fuel

Re-fuel after workouts with water and at least a piece of fruit if you're feeling hungry.

8. Don't Over Caffeinate.

Pre-workouts have caffeine and amphetamine-like compounds that can damage your blood vessels. Some of them have even been taken off the market because they've caused fatal heart conditions. Even just having coffee before a workout can be harmful. Caffeine restricts your blood vessels while you have blood pumping through them which can cause damage.

Strength Training Tips

1. Breathe

Before you start:
- Take some deep breaths with your nose and out of your mouth.
- Once you start your workout, breathe *out* through your nose as you lift the weight or contract the muscle.
- Breathe *in* through your nose as you lower the weight or extend the muscle.

2. Use Your Head

While you do the exercise, focus your mind on the muscle that you're trying to strengthen. It'll keep you focused during the workout and maximize the benefit. Your muscles respond to your thoughts. Studies have shown that even without *any* physical movement, it may seem crazy; strength is developed through mental attention to the muscle alone.

3. Increase Time Under Tension

The expression time under tension is basically how long your muscle is under strain during a set. Putting a muscle under strain for a long time causes more muscle breakdown.

In other words, slow down each set to 30-40 seconds each to increase muscle growth. Maintain a consistent tempo throughout the set, including the time that you're lowering the weight.

4. Rest

Your muscle must rest at least one day. And take at least one full rest day each week from exercise.

5. High Intensity Interval Training

If you hate putting the time in for cardio, then try high-intensity interval training. You'll burn the same number of calories in less time.

An example of HIIT on the elliptical or treadmill is:
- 4-minute walking warm-up
- 15 minutes of alternating between running for 45 seconds then walking for 45 seconds
- 4-minute walking cool- down

6. Aerobic Vs. Anaerobic

While there are many different forms of exercise, they can all be ultimately be lumped into either one of two categories: aerobic and anaerobic. No one particular kind of exercise is going to be better than the other. It just so happens that these two categories of exercise serve different purposes and impact the body differently. To learn more about the differences between aerobic and anaerobic exercise, read on further.

7. Aerobic

Aerobic fitness can also be considered cardiovascular fitness. Essentially, aerobic exercise is any moderately intense exercise that gets the heart rate up and increases the body's internal temperature. During aerobic exercise, there is moderate stress on the muscles and the heart. Typically, aerobic exercises are more sustainable. It is easier to sustain aerobic exercise for a prolonged duration when compared to anaerobic exercise.

When the body is in an aerobic state, the heart rate is raised to an uncomfortable state, but it isn't uncomfortable enough to the point that one wouldn't be able to talk anymore. Aerobic exercises are practical for weight loss because they induce calorie burn while you are performing the movements. Here are some examples of aerobic exercises:
- Running
- Swimming
- Jumping rope
- Brisk Walking
- Cycling
- Rowing

8. Anaerobic

Anaerobic exercises are generally more intense and can't be sustained for prolonged periods. Typically, these are composed of movements that are performed in short bursts at a rapid pace. When your body achieves an anaerobic state, your heart rate gets so high to the extent that you wouldn't be able to focus on anything else other than trying to breathe.

During anaerobic exercise, the lactic acid will gradually build up in your muscles and eventually lead to muscle failure or numbness. Anaerobic exercises are mostly associated with muscle growth and strength gains. This is how they differ from aerobic exercises that focus on stamina, endurance, and overall conditioning. Anaerobic exercises are practical for weight loss because they put the body's metabolism on hyperdrive for up to 48 hours after training.

Here are a few examples of anaerobic exercises:

- Olympic Weightlifting
- Sprinting
- High-Intensity Interval Training
- CrossFit
- Gymnastics
- Calisthenics

The 10 Components of Fitness

If you think that you can lose weight by being exceptionally good in just two or three fitness components, then that's fine. However, if you're intent is on understanding the science of exercise and how you can holistically approach your fitness training, then you need to acquaint yourself with every single one of these components.

1. Endurance

Endurance is the human body's ability to take in, process, and deliver oxygen. Whenever you engage in strenuous physical activity, your body will use more oxygen than is required than when you are merely at rest. So, the better endurance you have, the more your body will be able to keep up with you even as you keep pushing yourself with your training and exercise. To train your endurance, you need to engage in physical activity that elevates your heart rate to an uncomfortable state. Then, you need to maintain that elevated heart rate for as long as you can. The key to getting better every time is through gradual sensory overload. As your heart gets stronger, specific physical tasks get more comfortable. When that's the case, to make the heart even more robust, the physical task must become more challenging as well.

2. Stamina

Next comes stamina. Stamina is a lot like endurance in the sense that it has to do with the body's ability to sustain physical movement under pressure and tension. However, while regular endurance is concerned with cardiovascular strength, stamina has more to do with the muscles' endurance. The better your stamina is, the more efficient your body will be at breaking down energy sources like fat and glycogen.

So, to be more concrete about it, your endurance is going to be what enables you to run for two hours without stopping. Your stamina is going to be what enables you to sustain full-speed sprint intervals after a short period of rest. If you have good stamina, you will recover faster after a burst of energy expenditure.

3. Strength

Strength. While this is a word that many people might be familiar with, not too many are acquainted with its scientific definition. Your strength is the ability of your muscular units to apply force in a single contraction. When you build your strength, you can move more weight and apply more force through your muscles. Strength training is done by lifting heavy weights for numerous reps. This is an effective training method for fat loss because it demands so much from the body's metabolic system. At the same time, strength allows the human body to do more things during workouts.

4. Power

Strength and power are two components that are often intertwined with one another and that is because they share a few very fundamental principles. Strength is determined by the amount of force that your muscles can produce. However, your power is determined by the speed at which your muscles' generated force is applied. This is why power is a crucial component in workouts like Olympic weightlifting, sprinting, or boxing. When you are powerful, you can exert your strength at a much faster and more efficient rate. This translates to better athletic performance.

5. Agility

Think of a fly in your room that you are desperately trying to swat but just can't seem to. You see the fly moving towards a specific direction. In anticipation, you try to swat it, but they can swiftly transition towards another unexpected direction to catch you off guard.

This is agility. Your body can speedily transition from one movement pattern to another. In sports, boxers would be perfect examples of agility. A boxer's speed to block a punch from an opponent and speedily counter it with a punch of their own would be a showcase of their agility. However, to improve your agility, you also need to improve other components of fitness as well. These components are speed, coordination, accuracy, balance and flexibility. This will be discussed in-depth as we make our way further down this list.

6. Speed

Speed is your body's ability to reduce the amount of time necessary to cycle through a repeated movement. If we go back to the example of the boxer, a manifestation of that boxer's speed would be the number of punches that they would be able to throw within a given period repeatedly.

Naturally, other factors come into play here such as stamina and endurance. It's not uncommon for specific physical components of fitness to intertwine and complement one another. Speed can be manifested in different ways and is one of the most challenging fitness components to train.

7. Flexibility

When you think of flexibility, likely, you would automatically think of a yogi. Flexibility is your body's ability to maintain strength and control through different planes of range of motion. As you may already know, your body is made up of different joints and muscles. The more flexible you are, the better you will be at manipulating your body to get into certain positions without experiencing any pain or extreme discomfort. Flexibility is essential in training because it is a good indicator of how injury-prone an athlete might be. If you are not flexible, the more prone you are to injuries surrounding your joints and muscles. In other words, flexibility is your body's ability to bend without breaking.

8. Balance

Balance is all about control. One of the most important aspects of fitness is your body's ability to control its centre of gravity about its support base. Balance is an essential fitness component for athletes like skateboarders, skiers, surfers, gymnasts, martial artists and more. Balance is more classified under neurological fitness than physical fitness as a lot of it has to do with the brain's power to send signals to focal points of the body. However, while not many athletes notice it, balance plays a vital role in simplifying simple movements like running and jumping.

9. Coordination

Coordination is one's ability to maintain composure and control while simultaneously performing different movement patterns. For dancers, coordination is critical. While the left arm performs a particular movement pattern, a dancer must also master the art of having the right leg perform a different movement pattern. Like balance coordination is also classified under neurological fitness. It's something that can only be trained through sheer repetition and practice.

10.   Accuracy

Lastly, there is accuracy. To put it simply, accuracy is the body's ability to control one's movement with precision and direction at varying intensities. Accuracy is a component of fitness that is crucial for basketball players. For a basketball player's biomechanics to translate into a scored basket shooting the basketball is tantamount. And as you may have already guessed, accuracy is also a neurological skill, just like balance and coordination.

Benefits of Exercise

Yes, exercise is a powerful instrument that can be used to help you lose weight. More than just serving as a valuable tool for weight loss, however, regular exercise and physical activity will also provide you with other health benefits. Granted, not a lot of people would be too keen on the idea of several times a week getting sweaty and dirty from exercise. Some people will need something a little more compelling than others. Other benefits of exercising are listed below:

1. You'll have more energy

You can see some vast changes in your physical fitness whenever you work out daily. This partially means that your endurance and stamina are also going to improve. It is the duty of your stamina and toughness to have the energy to do the tasks you do every day. So, if you work out regularly, you will improve your job ability. You become more concentrated, inspired, empowered, and efficient in life when you have more energy. You are just going to start feeling like you have too much more motivation to do more things. For you to fulfil your aspirations and objectives, this energy would serve as power.

2. You Get Better Sleep at Night

Not many individuals know that having a decent night's sleep is one of the most important advantages of exercise. Care of this. Your body, as a human being, is still primed to produce a lot of energy to support itself. It expects you to have lots of tasks to do during the day, so it plans a range of energy to be taken up by you. There is a lot of pent-up energy inside them with certain inactive persons that does not get used up and remains with them until the night. This is how exercising will allow individuals to sleep well. You would be depleting the energy supplies the body generates when you consume that energy by engaging in intense physical exercise. This could translate to a greater amount of overnight sleep for you.

3. You Get an Endorphin Boost

For individuals who work out daily, endorphins, otherwise referred to as positive hormones, will still be in complete supply. Your brain activates the release of hormones called endorphins into the bloodstream while you work out. It is the duty of endorphins to improve your morale and make you feel lighter and more positive about life. So, you literally give yourself a normal boost on endorphins if you work out. You build a fun atmosphere for yourself. Therefore, it's such a smart thing to work out for individuals if they feel depressed, nervous or angry. For the disposition of a human the endorphin release will do wonders.

4. You Have Improved Sex Life

While sex is a very emotional (and maybe even spiritual) act for many people, it still has a significant physical component to it. When you have a thriving sex life, you will have to reach a certain degree of fitness. If you want to optimize the fun that you have in your bedroom, you need to have strength, agility, stamina and even versatility. These are all things you get better at whenever you consistently workout and practice. Sweat is often understood to be a natural aphrodisiac. In the bedroom, you have a lot to learn by doing work in the gym.

5. You More Comfortable with Yourself

Finally, you just end up feeling better about yourself after a workout. Sure, when you work out consistently, you are also chiselling your physique. The physical changes that will take place in your body will give you a renewed sense of confidence and self-esteem. On top of that, whenever you achieve certain fitness milestones, you become proud of that sense of achievement. Overall, you just end up being prouder of who you are as a person whenever you exercise. You become so much more comfortable and at ease with who you are.

You don't have to be a professional athlete to set goals for yourself. That's not necessary. The point here is to figure out how you can best accelerate your journey to lose weight. And the answer is for you to have a trustworthy and reliable training program that you enjoy doing and can sustain. That's the whole point. Sure, you can be proud of yourself for going out and running for an hour. However, if you don't enjoy running and you don't see the point in it, then it would be tough for you to sustain it as a training program.

The important thing here is that you understand why it's essential for you to exercise. You've merely been given the tools that you need to motivate yourself to start being more active. If you're still having trouble determining what kind of training routine would be best suited for you, don't worry.

Chapter 4: Food list – What is allowed and what is not

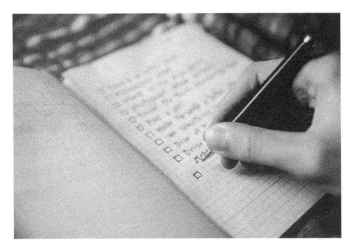

Many of the Optavia plans include its "supplies," like bars, smoothies, cookies, cereals and some savoury options, such as soup and mashed potatoes. These processed foods often list soy or whey protein as their first ingredient.

Lean, green meals complement the rest of the diet, which you purchase and prepare yourself.

These include:
- 5-7 ounces of cooked lean protein like egg white, chicken, fish, soy;
- 3 servings of non-starchy vegetables like cucumbers, lettuce, celery;
- 2 servings of healthy fats like olives, olive oil, avocado.

Based on the Optavia diet plan you choose; you will eat 2 to 5 pre-packaged replacement meals per day.

You will prepare and eat 1 to 3 of your low-calorie meals, which should be mostly lean protein and non-starchy vegetables.

While no food is technically prohibited in the diet, many (such as sweets) are discouraged.

- Free-range turkey (Always check the label and choose a lean turkey cut that complies with Optavia's guidelines for your sixth meal).
- Pumpkin seeds
- Put salt and pepper in to give it flavour. You can also mix pumpkin seeds in a salad.
- Grilled shrimp
- With this lean protein, you can create many varieties of meals. Thread a few skewers and arrange them on the grill or season the shrimp with Cajun spices and serve with grilled peppers and zucchini on the side.

- Cucumbers
- The Optavia diet requires non-starchy vegetables for the sixth daily meal.
- Cucumbers may work for you, or you can snack on celery sticks.
- Tuna

If you travel a lot, this light meal does not require any preparation time. Take a can of tuna and stir with freshly squeezed lemon juice, chopped celery, and olives.

Lean Meals

The "lean and green" meals you prepare should incorporate a 5 to 7 ounce serving of cooked lean protein.

Optavia differentiates between lean, leaner, and leanest protein sources.

I'll give you some examples to distinguish them:
- Lean: salmon, lamb or pork chops;
- Leaner: swordfish or chicken breast;
- Leanest: cod, shrimp and egg whites.

Green Meal

In Optavia's 5 & 1 program, you can add two non-starchy vegetables and protein to your lean and green meal.

Vegetables are broken down into lower, moderate, and higher carb categories, with the following examples:
- Low carb: green salad
- Moderate carbohydrates: cauliflower or summer squash
- Higher carbohydrates: broccoli or peppers
- Healthy fats

Beyond lean protein and non-starchy vegetables, a lean and green meal can be made with two servings of healthy fats like olive or nut oil, flax-seed, or avocado.

When people have achieved their desired weight loss through meal replacements, lean proteins, and non-starchy vegetables, they can switch to a plan to maintain their weight.

In Optavia's weight maintenance plans, users can start reintroducing other foods. Low-fat dairy, fruit and whole grains are incorporated in Optavia's 3 & 3 and 4 & 2 & 1 weight maintenance plans.

Foods/Nourishment to keep away from

Except for carbs in the pre-packaged Optavia "Fuelings", most carb-containing nourishments and refreshments are restricted while on the 5&1 Plan. Certain fats are additionally limited, just like every seared food.

Nourishments to stay away from — except if remembered for the Fueling — include:

- Fried foods/nourishments: meats, fish, shellfish, vegetables, desserts like baked goods
- Refined grains: white bread, pasta, scones, flapjacks, flour tortillas, saltines, white rice, treats, cakes, baked goods
- Certain fats: margarine, coconut oil, muscular shortening
- Whole fat dairy: milk, cheddar, yogurt
- Alcohol: all assortments
- Sugar-improved refreshments: pop, natural product juice, sports drinks, caffeinated drinks, sweet tea

The accompanying nourishments are untouchable while on the 5&1 Plan yet included back during the 6-week progress stage and permitted during the 3&3 Plan:

- Fruit: all-new natural product
- Low fat or without fat dairy: yogurt, milk, cheddar
- Whole grains: entire grain bread, high fiber breakfast oat, earthy colored rice, entire wheat pasta
- Legumes: peas, lentils, beans, soybeans
- Starchy vegetables: yams, white potatoes, corn, peas

During the Change Stage and 3&3 Plan, you're particularly urged to eat berries over different natural products, as they're lower in carbs.

Chapter 5: Which is the Perfect Plan for You?

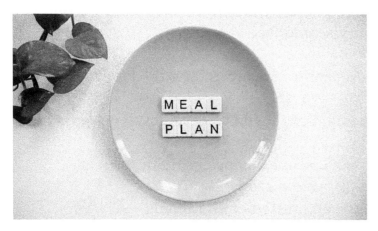

Choosing the perfect Plan is simple when you understand your health and wellness needs. The truth is that not everybody desires to lose excessive amounts of weight. Sometimes, people go on a diet to maintain a healthy mind and body. The one thing that dieters don't have to be worried about is missing their favorite dishes and foods they used to enjoy. While the Optavia diet promotes a low-calorie diet, I could still prepare mouth-watering foods at home. With the Optavia diet, I am regularly eating throughout the day. The diet advises eating six or seven times per day (about every two to three hours) depending on the specific plan you choose. There are three customized low-calories plans to choose from depending on your personal weight loss goal.

For instance:
1. the 5-and-1 Plan is suitable for those who desire to lose a considerable amount of weight in the shortest amount of time.
2. the 4-and-2and-1 Plan offers more flexibility.
3. the 3-and-3 Plan is excellent for maintaining weight loss.

Below is a more in-depth look into each Plan:

The 5-and-1 Plan
Average price: $392.15 for 119 servings.
The Optavia 5-and-1 plan requires dieters to eat six small meals a day. This healthy eating habit promotes weight loss and ensures that dieters have sufficient energy throughout the day. Five out of the six meals consist of Optavia "Fuelings". There are over sixty delicious "Fuelings" to choose from that are ready-made, convenient, and packed with nutrients. The friendly and helpful Optavia health coaches are available to guide dieters on the best selection of "Fuelings" to choose from for a varied diet plan. The sixth meal of the day is a homemade meal using the "Lean and Green" meal guidelines. Preparing my healthy meals allowed me to recognize what optimal Nutrition looks like and soon eating healthy became second nature.

The 4-and-2-and-1 Plan
Average price: $399 for 140 servings

A 4-and-2-and-1 plan is an excellent option for those who prefer a less stringent diet and more flexible meal plans to reach their weight loss goals. The Plan is most suitable for those who:

- Want to continue incorporating all of the food groups (including fruits, dairy, and starches) in their meals
- Have type 1 diabetes and are closely supervised by a healthcare provider
- Have type 2 diabetes
- They are sixty-five years or older and rarely engage in exercise or similar activities
- Have less than fifteen pounds (6.8 kilograms) of weight to lose.

This meal plan works similarly to the 5-and-1 meal plan; however, the ratios are different. In this Plan, dieters would eat four "Fuelings", two "Lean and Green" homemade meals, and one healthy snack. Dieters would still be required to eat six times per day or every two to three hours. Some of the Optavia-approved snacks that I love to munch on include puffed sweet and salty snacks, puffed ranch snacks, olive oil and sea salt popcorn and sharp cheddar and sour cream popcorn. Sometimes, I prefer making my homemade snacks instead, allowing me to practice my culinary skills. On the 4-and-2-and-1 plan, I can consume one starch, fruit, or dairy snack a day. Below are a few examples of servings for each type of snack:

Starch Snacks

- One slice of whole grain bread
- 3/4 cups of cold whole-grain cereal (such as bran flakes or oats)
- 1/2 cup of cooked cereal
- 1/2 cup of corn or peas
- 1 cup of winter squash
- 1/4 large (3 ounces) baked potato
- 1/3 cup of cooked brown rice
- 1/2 cup of cooked legumes like beans or lentils

Fruit Snacks

- One small piece (4 ounces) of fresh fruit like an apple, pear, or orange
- 1/2 cup of frozen fruit
- 1 cup of fresh, cubed melon like cantaloupe or honeydew
- 3/4 cup of fresh berries
- 1/2 cup of canned fruit like peaches, pineapples, or fruit cocktail (opt for fruit canned in water and not syrup)
- 17 fresh grapes
- 1/2 large grapefruit

Dairy Snacks

- 3/4 cups (6 ounces) of low-fat yogurt
- 1 cup of unsweetened low-fat or fat-free milk (opt for almond, cashew, or soy milk)
- 1/2 cup of fat-free evaporated milk

The 3-and-3 Plan

Average price: $309.55 for 130 servings

One of the quickest lessons I learned early in the Optavia Diet is that losing weight is more than just seeing the number drop on a scale. Weight loss is a journey, and that once I had reached my weight loss goal, I had to continue on the path of optimal health. This means that I had to maintain my weight loss and continue eating healthily. The 3-and-3 Plan helped me sustain my healthy weight and maintain all of the good habits I had learned along the way. It is an excellent plan for dieters to transition to once all of their weight loss goals have been met, and healthy living becomes a lifestyle. The significant difference between the 4-and-2-and-1 Plan and the 3-and-3 Plan is that the latter incorporates more food choices in the correct portion sizes. With this, I could eat three Optavia "Fuelings" and three "Lean and Green" balanced meals per day (every two to three hours). To get started with this Plan, I had to follow three simple steps:

- **Step 1**: Calculate my Total Energy Expenditure (TEE). This is the number of calories I burn per day.
- **Step 2**: Choosing my meal plan based on my TEE. There were various meal plans for me to choose from, ranging from 1,200 to 2,500 calories per day.

- **Step 3**: Familiarizing myself with my meal plan's food groups. Since the 3- and-3 Plan is a maintenance plan, I could eat a lot more foods such as fruits, dairy, starch, protein, fats, and vegetables.

Chapter 6: The 30-Day Rapid Weight Loss Program Challenge

Day	Breakfast	Lunch	Dinner	Dessert
1	Overnight oats	Thai noodle salad	Buddha Bowl with seitan	Fresh fruit bowl
2	Overnight oats	Thai noodle salad	Creamy garlic & lemon alfredo	Fresh fruit bowl
3	Scrambled tofu & toast	Crunchy veggie wrap with tofu	Southwest stuffed peppers	Oatmeal cookies
4	Scrambled tofu & toast	Crispy veggie wrap with tofu	Chickpea noodle soup	Oatmeal cookies
5	Cinnamon Quinoa Bowl	Chickpea noodle soup (leftover)	Buddha bowl with tempeh	Oatmeal cookies
6	Ultimate Breakfast Burrito	Blackbean taco salad	Vegan pizza	No-bake brownies
7	Fluffy Vegan Pancakes	VBLT	Party Friendly pho	No-bake brownies
8	Overnight oats— Option 2	Middle East chickpea wrap	Buddha bowl with tofu	No-bake brownies
9	Overnight oats— Option 2	Middle East chickpea wrap	Creamy garlic & lemon alfredo	Fresh fruit bowl
10	Scrambled tofu in a wrap	Curried tofu salad	Southwest stuffed peppers	Fresh fruit bowl
11	Scrambled tofu in a wrap	Curried tofu salad	Creamy tomato & basil soup	Chocolate peanut butter fudge
12	Chocolate Quinoa Bowl	Creamy tomato & basil soup	Buddha bowl with peanut tofu	Chocolate peanut butter fudge

13	Sweet Potato Tempeh hash	Crunchy veggie wrap	Vegan pizza	Chocolate peanut butter fudge
14	Fluffy Vegan pancakes	VBLT	Mexican lentil soup	Apple crisp
15	Overnight oats— Option 3	Mexican lentil soup (leftover)	Southwest stuffed peppers	Apple crisp
16	Overnight oats— Option 3	Curried tofu wrap	Party friendly pho	Oatmeal cookies
17	Scrambled tofu & a bagel	Curried tofu wrap	Creamy garlic & lemon alfredo	Oatmeal cookies
18	Scrambled tofu & a bagel	Crunchy veggie wrap	Buddha bowl with tempeh	Fresh fruit bowl
19	Cinnamon Quinoa Bowl	Thai noodle salad	VBLT	Fresh fruit bowl
20	Ultimate Breakfast Burrito	Blackbean taco salad	Creamy tomato & basil soup	No-bake brownies
21	Fluffy Vegan Pancakes	VBLT & tomato soup (leftover)	Vegan pizza	No-bake brownies
22	Overnight oats— Option 1	Middle East chickpea salad	Buddha bowl with seitan	No-bake brownies
23	Overnight oats— Option 1	Middle East chickpea salad	Creamy garlic & lemon alfredo	Fresh fruit bowl
24	Scrambled tofu & roasted potatoes	Crunchy veggie wrap	Chickpea noodle soup	Fresh fruit bowl
25	Scrambled tofu & roasted potatoes	Chickpea noodle soup (leftover)	Southwest stuffed peppers	Chocolate peanut butter fudge
26	Chocolate Quinoa Bowl	Blackbean taco salad	Buddha bowl with peanut tofu	Chocolate peanut butter fudge
27	Sweet Potato Tempeh hash	Curried tofu wrap	Creamy garlic & lemon alfredo	Chocolate peanut butter fudge

28	Ultimate Breakfast Burrito	VBLT	Party friendly pho	Apple crisp
29	Fluffy Vegan Pancakes	Mexican lentil soup	Vegan Pizza	Apple crisp
30	Overnight oats	Creamy tomato & basil soup	Southwest stuffed peppers	Fresh fruit bowl

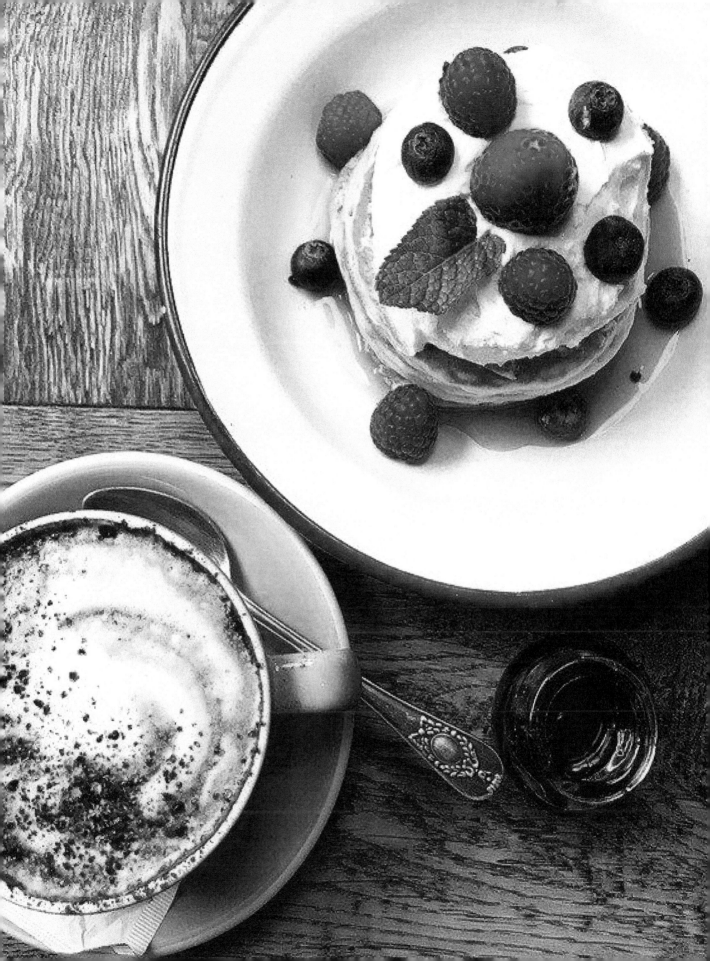

Chapter 7: Breakfast Recipes

Breakfast One - Breakfast Hash

Nutritional Information Per Serving:

280 Calories, 10 grams of Fat, 36 grams of Carbs, 6 grams of Protein

Time: 20 minutes

Serving Size: 3 servings

Ingredients:

- 3 medium potatoes, diced
- 1 cup onion, chopped
- 1 medium red bell pepper, chopped
- 1 cups mushrooms, sliced
- 1 teaspoon spices of choice (garlic, cumin, paprika, or combo)
- 2 tablespoons avocado oil
- Himalayan salt and pepper to preference

Directions:

1. In a medium skillet, pour and mix avocado oil and potatoes.
2. Sauté on medium heat until potatoes are soft or slightly crispy.
3. Add in other vegetables and spices.
4. Sauté until vegetables are soft.

Breakfast Two - Breakfast Cookies

Nutritional Information Per Cookie: 207 Calories, 12 grams of fat, 24 grams of carbs, 5 grams of protein

Time: 15 minutes

Serving Size: 8 cookies

Ingredients:

- 1 cup old fashioned rolled oats
- ½ cup oat flour
- ½ cup dried cranberries
- ½ cup pepitas, unsalted
- ¼ cup ground flax seed
- 1 tablespoon of chia seeds
- 1 teaspoon cinnamon
- ½ teaspoon baking powder
- generous pinch of Himalayan salt
- 1 large banana, mashed
- 3 tablespoons melted coconut oil
- 2 tablespoons almond milk, unsweetened

Directions:

1. Preheat oven to 375 Fahrenheit or 190 degrees Celsius. Line a baking sheet with parchment paper.
2. Combine all dry ingredients in a large mixing bowl and mix well.
3. Stir in banana, coconut oil, and almond milk.
4. Let the mixture sit for 5 minutes.
5. Start scooping the mixture and form a small ball. Place ball on lined baking sheet and press to flatten into cookies.
6. Bake for 16 minutes or until the edges of the cookies are golden.

Breakfast Three - Protein Shake: Vanilla Cashew

Nutritional Information Per Serving: 450 Calories, 26 grams of Fat, 45 grams of Carbs, 15 grams of Protein

Time: 5 minutes

Serving Size: 1 serving

Ingredients:

- 1 banana
- ¼ cup raw cashews
- 1 cup almond milk, unsweetened
- 1 tablespoon cashew butter (or peanut butter)
- 1 tablespoon of chia seeds
- ½ teaspoon vanilla extract
- ½ cup ice cubes

Directions:

1. Place all ingredients in a high-powered blender and blend until smooth.

Breakfast Four - Zucchini Pancakes

Nutritional Information Per Serving: 192 Calories, 7 grams of Fat, 24 grams of Carbs, 7 grams of Protein

Time: 12 minutes

Serving Size: 2 servings

Ingredients:

- ½ cup chickpea flour, sifted/lump free
- ½ cup water
- 3 teaspoons avocado oil
- 2 cups zucchini, coarsely grated
- Himalayan salt and black pepper to preference

Directions:

1. In a medium bowl, mix flour, water, salt, salt, pepper, and 1 teaspoon of avocado oil. Mix until smooth or until the batter has no lumps.
2. Add in zucchini. Stir.
3. Add 1 teaspoon of oil in a nonstick skillet and warm over medium heat. Pour in half of the batter and cook for five minutes.

4. Carefully flip the pancake and cook for an additional four minutes or until the center appears golden brown.
5. Follow steps three and four to cook the remaining pancake.

Breakfast Five - High Protein Pudding

Nutritional Information Per Serving: 455 Calories, 24 grams of Fat, 53 grams of Carbs, 55 grams of Protein

Time: 5 minutes prep, (overnight recipe)

Serving Size: 2 servings

Ingredients:

- ½ cup buckwheat groats, dry
- 2 scoops vegan pea protein powder
- 1 banana
- ½ cup oat milk
- 2 tablespoons natural almond butter (substitute a different nut butter if preferred)
- 2 teaspoons cinnamon (optional)

Directions:

1. Add the groats to a bowl and cover with water. Soak the oats overnight.
2. Use a strainer to remove water.
3. Place all ingredients, including the groats, in a high-speed blender and blend until smooth.
4. Serve immediately and add additional toppings if desired.

Nutritional Information Per Taco: 166 Calories, 23 grams of Fat, 20 grams of Carbs, 10 grams of Protein

Time: 10 minutes

Serving Size: 4 tacos

Ingredients:

Taco Ingredients:
- ½ cup black beans, (no salt added/low sodium)
- ½ cup salsa
- ½ medium avocado
- 4 corn tortillas

For the Eggs:
- 6 ounces block tofu, firm and drained
- ½ tablespoon olive oil
- ½ teaspoon turmeric
- 1 tablespoon nutritional yeast
- 1 tablespoon water
- sea salt and black pepper to preference

Directions:

1. To prepare the tofu eggs, pour olive oil into a skillet and warm over medium heat for one minute.
2. Add the tofu the skillet and mash into crumbles using a spatula.
3. Stir and cook tofu for 5 minutes or until most of the water is gone.
4. Add the remaining tofu ingredients and stir.
5. Prepare the tacos using the taco ingredients and tofu eggs.

Nutritional Information Per Muffin: 218 Calories, 7 grams of Fat, 34 grams of Carbs, 4 grams of Protein

Time: 35 minutes

Serving Size: 12 muffins

Ingredients:

- 1 ¼ cup almond milk, unsweetened
- 1 teaspoon apple cider vinegar
- 2 cups whole wheat pastry flour
- 2 tablespoons Stevia powder (2 teaspoons Stevia drops)
- 2 teaspoons baking powder
- 1 tablespoon cornstarch
- ⅓ cup melted coconut oil
- 1 teaspoon vanilla extract
- 1½ cups blueberries

Directions:

1. Preheat oven to 400 Fahrenheit or 205 Celsius. Line muffin pan with liners and lightly spray them with oil.
2. Combine almond milk and apple cider vinegar in a cup and set aside.
3. In a large mixing bowl, combine and mix all dry ingredients. Pour in the almond milk and apple cider vinegar mixture.
4. Add coconut oil and vinegar to the large mixing bowl.
5. Fold in blueberries.
6. Divide mixture evenly into the 12 liners.
7. Bake for 20-25 minutes or until the top is golden brown. Use a toothpick and wait to remove muffins until it comes out clean after being placed in the center.
8. Allow cooling and use an airtight container to store in the refrigerator or freezer.

Nutritional Information Per Serving: 410 Calories, 21 grams of Fat, 58 grams of Carbs, 4 grams of Protein

Time: 5 minutes

Serving Size: 1 serving

Ingredients:

- 1 medium sized banana
- 2 cups of fresh spinach
- ½ avocado
- 2 cups coconut milk, unsweetened
- 1 medium sized apple (remove core)
- 1 cup of ice
- cold water as needed/to preference

Directions:

1. Add all ingredients to a high-powered blender and blend until smooth.

Breakfast Nine - Bread Recipe, One

Nutritional Information Per Serving: 191 Calories, 12 grams of Fat, 16 grams of Carbs, 6 grams of Protein

Time: 1 hour 15 minutes

Serving Size: 15 servings

Ingredients:

- 2 cups rolled oats
- 5 tablespoons psyllium husks
- 1 cup sunflower seeds

- 2 tablespoons pepitas
- 2 tablespoons almonds, whole
- 2 tablespoons hazelnuts, whole
- ½ cup and 1 tablespoon ground flax seeds
- 2½ tablespoons chia seeds
- ½ teaspoon Himalayan salt
- 1½ teaspoon coconut oil
- 1¾ cups warm water

Directions:

1. In a large bowl, combine all ingredients. Mix well.
2. Cover the mixing bowl and refrigerate overnight.
3. When ready to bake, preheat oven to 390 Fahrenheit or 200 Celsius.
4. Grease a loaf pan with addition oil of your choice before pouring the batter into the loaf pan.
5. Once the batter is in the loaf pan, shape the dough to resemble a smooth, curved top.
6. Bake the bread for 50 minutes or up until an hour. Remove the pan and remove the loaf right away.

Breakfast Ten - Eggs and Toast

Nutritional Information Per Serving (Eggs): 100 Calories, 8 grams of Fat, 3 grams of Carbs, 12 grams of Protein

Time: 7-8 minutes

Serving Size: 3 servings

Ingredients:

For the Eggs:
- 15 oz firm tofu, drained
- ½ teaspoon onion powder
- ½ teaspoon garlic powder
- ¼ teaspoon turmeric powder

- 1 tablespoon nutritional yeast
- 1 tablespoon almond milk
- Himalayan salt and black pepper to preference

For the Toast:
- Toast vegan store-bought bread or bake homemade bread using the instructions from *Breakfast Nine*.

Directions:

1. In a non-stick skillet add all egg ingredients and sauté over medium heat. Use a spatula to break up the tofu into scramble-like pieces. This step should take about five to six minutes.
2. Serve the eggs with toast or any other additional vegan toppings.

Breakfast Eleven - Chickpea Skillet

Nutritional Information Per Serving: 425 Calories, 30 grams of Fat, 45 grams of Carbs, 19 grams of Protein

Time: 20 minutes

Serving Size: 2 servings

Ingredients:

- 2 medium potatoes, diced
- 2 tablespoons olive oil
- ½ teaspoon garlic powder
- 1 bell pepper, diced
- 1 small red onion, diced
- ½ cup chickpeas, drained and rinsed
- 1 handful fresh baby spinach
- 1 avocado, pitted and sliced
- 1 medium tomatoes, diced
- sea salt and black pepper to preference

Directions:

1. In a large pot, bring water to a boil. Add in potatoes and cook for 5 minutes. Drain potatoes.
2. In a cast iron skillet, heat olive oil over medium heat.
3. Add potatoes and spices to the skillet and spread the potatoes evenly. Do not stir for at least 5 minutes.
4. After five minutes, stir potatoes. Then spread them evenly across the pan again. Leave them for another five minutes or until crispy.
5. Add chopped bell pepper, chickpeas, and onion to the skillet. Cook until peppers are soft, then add in the spinach.
6. Stir the mixture and allow the spinach to soften for one minute. Then serve with toppings.

Breakfast Twelve - Chocolate Overnight Oats

Nutritional Information Per Serving: 430 Calories, 27 grams of Fat, 45 grams of Carbs, 10 grams of Protein

Time: 5 minutes, (overnight recipe)

Serving Size: 1 serving

Ingredients:

- ½ cup rolled oats
- 1 tablespoon cocoa powder, unsweetened
- 1 tablespoon of chia seeds
- 1 tablespoon coconut oil, melted
- ½ cup coconut milk
- 1 tablespoon vegan chocolate chips
- vegan sweetener of choice

Directions:

1. In a glass mason jar, combine all ingredients before giving a vigorous shake.
2. Place in the refrigerator overnight and enjoy the next morning!

Nutritional Information Per Serving: 545 Calories, 33 grams of Fat, 58 grams of Carbs, 10 grams of Protein

Time: 5 minutes

Serving Size: 1 serving

Ingredients:

For the Smoothie:
- ½ avocado
- 1 tablespoon cocoa powder, unsweetened
- 1 teaspoon vanilla extract
- ½ cup coconut milk, unsweetened
- ½ cup ice

For the Toppings:
- ¼ cup almonds, sliced
- 1 tablespoon vegan chocolate chips
- ¼ cup blueberries

Directions:

1. Add all smoothie ingredients to a high-powered blender and blend until smooth. Create a thick, icy consistency.
2. Pour into a wide bowl.
2. Sprinkle toppings on top of the smoothie and eat with a spoon.

Breakfast Fourteen - Peanut Butter Toast

Nutritional Information Per Serving: 540 Calories, 32 grams of Fat, 55 grams of Carbs, 16 grams of Protein

Time: 5 minutes

Serving Size: 1 serving

Ingredients:

- 1 slice of vegan bread (see bread recipe, *breakfast nine*)
- 2 tablespoons natural peanut butter
- 1 banana, sliced
- 1 tablespoons chia seeds

Directions:

1. Prepare the toast or bread by heating or placing it in the toaster.
2. Spread the nut butter on the toast and top with sliced banana, and chia seeds.

Breakfast Fifteen- Light Breakfast, Zero Prep

Nutritional Information Per Serving: 267 Calories, 15 grams of Fat, 32 grams of Carbs, 8 grams of Protein

Time: 1 minute

Serving Size: 1 serving

Ingredients:

- 23 almonds (one serving)
- 1 banana

Directions:

1. Grab these two items on the go when mornings are too busy to cook. Both items are extremely nutritious and will curb cravings until lunch time.

Nutritional Information Per Serving: 92.5 Calories, 1 grams of Fat, 53 grams of Carbs, 21 grams of Protein

Time: 10 minutes

Serving Size: 4 servings

Ingredients:

- ½ cup plain white flour
- ¼ cup vegan protein powder
- 1 tablespoon baking powder
- 2 tablespoons maple syrup
- 1 cup water
- pinch of Himalayan salt

Directions:

1. Mix all dry ingredients in a bowl.
2. Add maple syrup and stir.
3. Slowly add in water until batter is thick and lumpy.
4. In a skillet, add a drop of oil over medium-low heat and pour a small amount of batter into the pan.
5. Flip the pancake once bubbles appear and cook the other side for about one minute.
6. Repeat steps four and five until no batter remains.
7. Serve immediately with additional fruit or veggie toppings if desired.

Breakfast Seventeen - Egg Muffins

Nutritional Information Per Serving: 94 Calories, 4 grams of Fat, 6 grams of Carbs, 8.6 grams of Protein

Time: 45 minutes

Serving Size: 6 servings

Ingredients:

- 15 oz tofu, medium firm
- 2 teaspoons tahini
- 2 tablespoons chickpea flour
- 3 tablespoons nutritional yeast
- ¼ teaspoon turmeric
- ½ teaspoon onion powder
- 3 garlic cloves, finely chopped
- 1 cup broccoli, chopped
- 1 red bell pepper, chopped
- ½ cup corn

Directions:

1. Preheat oven to 350 Fahrenheit or 177 Celsius. Line muffin pan with 6 liners.
2. Over medium heat, add a small amount of olive oil to dry garlic. Add in broccoli, bell pepper, and corn.
3. After the vegetables have softened, add in the scallion and simmer for one minute. Remove vegetables from heat.
4. In a food processor or blender add in tofu, chickpea flour, nutritional yeast, tahini, turmeric, onion powder, salt, and pepper.
5. In a large bowl, combine vegetables and tofu mixture.
6. Distribute evenly into six muffin liners.
7. Bake for 25 to 35 minutes or until the tops are golden brown. Remove and allow cooling.

Breakfast Eighteen - Granola Cereal

Nutritional Information Per Serving: 241 Calories, 12 grams of Fat, 28 grams of Carbs, 6 grams of Protein

Time: 30 minutes

Serving Size: 4 servings

Ingredients:

- 1 cup rolled oats
- ⅓ cup pecans
- ½ teaspoon cinnamon
- 2 tablespoons natural almond butter
- ¼ cup maple syrup

Directions:

1. Preheat oven to 300 degrees Fahrenheit or 150 Celsius.
2. In a food processor place half of the oats and all of the pecans. Blend until a coarse flour appears. The mixture does not have to be smooth and can contain larger pecan pieces.
3. Combine the rest of the dry ingredients and add in the pecan oat flour.
4. Mix in the almond butter and syrup. Stir well.
5. Place the granola onto a baking sheet and bake for 25-30 minutes or until the mixture is crisp.
6. Remove and allow cooling before storing in an airtight container.
7. For breakfast, consume the cereal with a vegan milk and add in fruit of your choice if desired.

Breakfast Nineteen - Strawberry Banana Smoothie

Nutritional Information Per Serving: 255 Calories, 17 grams of Fat, 12 grams of Carbs, 14 grams of Protein

Time: 5 minutes

Serving Size: 4 servings

Ingredients:

- 10 strawberries, frozen
- 1 large banana, frozen
- 1 cup coconut milk, unsweetened

- ¾ cup hemp seeds
- ½ teaspoon vanilla extract

Directions:

1. Place all ingredients into a high-powered blender and blend until smooth. Use more coconut milk or water as needed.

Breakfast Twenty - Lemon Doughnuts

Nutritional Information Per Serving: 120 Calories, 5 grams of Fat, 23 grams of Carbs, 6 grams of Protein

Time: 35 minutes

Serving Size: 6 servings/doughnuts

Ingredients:

- 1½ cups all-purpose flour
- 1 teaspoon baking powder
- 2 tablespoons ground flax seed
- 6 tablespoons water
- ½ teaspoon powdered Stevia
- 4 teaspoons poppy seeds
- 1 tablespoon lemon juice
- 1 medium lemon, zested
- 1 teaspoon vanilla extract
- 6 tablespoons coconut milk

Directions:

1. Preheat oven to 375 Fahrenheit or 190 degrees Celsius. Grease a non-stick doughnut pan.
2. Mix the ground flax seed and water in a small cup and place the mixture in the refrigerator for 20 minutes.
3. Meanwhile, in a large bowl, mix all the ingredients together until well blended. The ingredients should turn into a thick batter.

4. Add the flax and water mixture.
5. Spoon the batter into the doughnut pan and smooth the top.
6. Bake the doughnuts for 10 to 12 minutes.
7. Remove the pan and allow cooling before storing or consuming.

Breakfast Twenty-One- Cream Cheese Recipe

Nutritional Information Per Serving: 350 Calories, 11 grams of Fat, 5 grams of Carbs, 3 grams of Protein

Time: 5 minutes (overnight recipe)

Serving Size: 6 servings

Ingredients:

- ⅜ cup cashews, raw
- 1 tablespoon olive oil
- 1 teaspoon garlic, minced
- 1 tablespoon lemon juice
- ½ teaspoon apple cider vinegar
- 1 teaspoon oregano
- Himalayan salt and black pepper to taste

Directions:

1. Place cashews in hot water and soak for one hour if you have a powerful blender, or soak them overnight.
2. Drain cashews and add to blender with the rest of the listed ingredients.
3. Blend until mixture has the consistency of a creamy paste. Add a dab of warm water if needed.
4. Serve with a vegan bagel, or over toast with your favorite toppings.

Breakfast Twenty-Two- Breakfast Sweet Potatoes

Nutritional Information Per Serving: 460 Calories, 11 grams of Fat, 60 grams of Carbs, 8 grams of Protein

Time: 55 minutes

Serving Size: 2 servings

Ingredients:

- 2 medium sweet potatoes
- 1 large banana, sliced
- ½ cup blueberries
- 1 tablespoons chia seeds
- 4 tablespoons natural almond butter
- 2 tablespoons maple syrup

Directions:

1. Preheat oven to 400 Fahrenheit or 205 Celsius.
2. Place sweet potatoes directly on the rack and bake for 45 minutes or until soft.
3. Cut the sweet potato in half and split the above toppings between the two.
4. Serve immediately or warm up the sweet potatoes when ready to consume.

Breakfast Twenty-Three- Chia Pudding

Nutritional Information Per Serving: 435 Calories, 20 grams of Fat, 47 grams of Carbs, 15 grams of Protein

Time: 5 minutes, (overnight recipe)

Serving Size: 1 serving

Ingredients:

- ¼ cup cooked quinoa

- 2 tablespoons chia seeds
- 3 tablespoons hemp hearts
- ½ teaspoon vanilla extract
- 2 tablespoon maple syrup
- ¾ cup coconut milk

Directions:

1. Add all ingredients to a glass mason jar and shake vigorously.
2. Place in refrigerator to soak for at least two hours, or overnight.
3. Remove when ready to consume and top with additional fruit or toppings as desired.

Breakfast Twenty-Four- Cheesy Casserole

Nutritional Information Per Serving: 205 Calories, 5 grams of Fat, 34 grams of Carbs, 8 grams of Protein

Time: 1 hour

Serving Size: 8 servings

Ingredients:

For the Casserole:
- 4 cups shredded potatoes (store bought or freshly grated)
- ¾ cup onions, diced
- ½ cup red bell pepper, chopped
- ¾ cup fresh spinach
- ¼ cup nutritional yeast
- Himalayan salt and pepper to preference

For the Sauce:
- 1 cup potatoes, peeled and diced
- ¼ cup carrots, diced
- ¼ cup onions, diced
- 1 cup almond milk

- ½ cup raw cashews
- 4 tablespoons nutritional yeast
- 1 tablespoon lemon juice
- ½ teaspoon garlic powder

Directions:

For the Sauce:
1. In a medium-sized pot, boil 3 cups of water. Add potatoes, carrots, and onions. Cook until tender or for 15 minutes.
2. Drain the vegetables when finished and place into blender along with all other cheese sauce ingredients.
3. Blend until smooth.

For the Casserole:
4. Preheat oven to 350 Fahrenheit or 177 Celsius. Line a baking dish with parchment paper.
5. In a large bowl mix onion, red bell peppers, shredded potatoes, cheese sauce, and spices.
6. Add in spinach leaves and mix again.
7. Add mixture to the dish and bake for 30 minutes. Remove and serve warm.

Breakfast Twenty-Five - French Toast

Nutritional Information Per Serving: 222 Calories, 12 grams of Fat, 25 grams of Carbs, 4 grams of Protein

Time: 30 minutes

Serving Size: 4 serving

Ingredients:

- 1 large banana
- ¾ cup full-fat coconut milk
- 1 tablespoon maple syrup
- 1 teaspoon vanilla extract

- ½ teaspoon cinnamon
- 1 tablespoon coconut oil
- 4-6 slices bread of choice

Directions:

1. Add the banana, coconut milk, maple syrup, vanilla, and cinnamon to a blender. Blend until smooth.
2. Pour mixture into a large bowl that will be suitable for dipping the bread.
3. In a skillet, heat a small amount of coconut oil over medium heat. Use oil only as needed to prevent burning.
4. Dip the bread into the mixture and coat both sides. Place into the frying pan.
5. Cook the bread on each side for a few minutes or until golden brown.
6. Serve with additional toppings of choice.

Breakfast Twenty-Six - Overnight Oats

Nutritional information per serving:

Calories	260	Carbs	36g	Iron	15%
Sugar	3g	Protein	11g	Calcium	18%
Fiber	13g	Fat	6g		

What You Need:

- Dairy-free milk (0.5 cup or 120ml)
- Rolled oats (0.5 cup or 45g)
- Chia seeds (0.75 tbsp or 9g)

What to Do:

1. Add to a mason jar or any container with a lid, the dairy-free milk, chia seeds, and the optional flavors listed below. Stir with a spoon to gently

combine; ingredients do not have to be completely mixed with the dairy-free milk.
2. Add the oats and stir gently again. Use a spoon to press down the oats, make sure they are entirely covered by the dairy-free milk and secure with a lid or cover. Let rest in the fridge overnight.
3. To prepare them the next day, you can enjoy them cold, or you can warm them for approx. sixty seconds in the microwave. You can also add more toppings as a garnish.

Breakfast Twenty-Seven - Scrambled Tofu

Nutritional information per serving:

Calories	212	Carbs	7g	Sodium	20%
Sugar	3g	Protein	16g	Calcium	40%
Fiber	2g	Fat	15g		

What You Need:

Scramble:

- Extra-firm tofu - 8 ounces (227g)
- Olive oil - 1-2 tbsp (15-30ml)
- Veggies, chopped (see ideas below)

Sauce:
- Sea salt - 1 tsp (5g)
- Cumin powder - 1 tsp (5g)
- Garlic powder - 1 tsp (5g)
- Onion powder - 1 tsp (5g)
- Water, as needed

What to Do:

1. Remove tofu from package, drain the water and pat the tofu dry. Wrap tofu in an absorbent towel (paper towel or a clean dishcloth) and rest something heavy on top for ten to fifteen minutes. This process is called "pressing," and it removes excess water from tofu. This process allows the flavor of your meal to be more pronounced.

2. While the tofu is being pressed, mix the sauce by adding all the dry spices to a bowl and add water in small portions—1-2 tbsp (15-30ml) at a time to make a pourable sauce. Mix and set aside.

3. Prep the selection of veggies, once everything is chopped preheat over medium heat, a medium-sized skillet. Once hot, add olive oil and for one to two minutes sauté the hard vegetables. If using kale, spinach, or other leafy greens wait until the other veggies have softened, approximately five minutes, then add the greens and sauté for two to four minutes. Season with a dash of salt and pepper while cooking.

4. While the veggies cook, unwrap the pressed tofu and in a bowl, crumble the tofu into small pieces to resemble the look of scrambled eggs.

5. Push the veggies over to one side of the skillet and add the tofu to the open space. Sauté the tofu for two minutes. Stir the prepared sauce again and pour most of it over the tofu, with the remainder to be saved and drizzled over the veggies. Stir everything together in the pan quickly and cook for five to seven minutes until you see the tofu browning slightly. Some should be crispy but leave most of it softly cooked.

6. Serve immediately or save for meal prep, giving you breakfast options for a few days. This recipe can be doubled, or even tripled and left in the freezer for up to one month, reheating on a stovetop and adding even more flavor at that time.

Nutritional information per serving:

Calories	236	Carbs	40g	Iron	40%
Sugar	9g	Protein	8g	Magnesium	20%
Fiber	4g	Fat	6g		

What You Need:

- Uncooked white quinoa - 1 cup (172g)
- Non-dairy milk (unsweetened) - 1 cup (236ml)
- Canned coconut milk - 1 cup (236ml). Choose the lite option for less fat
- Cocoa powder (unsweetened) - 1 tbsp (15g)
- Maple syrup - 2 tbsp (30ml)
- Vanilla extract - 1 tsp (5ml)
- Pinch of salt
- Toppings of your choice (see below)

What to Do:

1. In a fine, mesh strainer, rinse the quinoa for two minutes. As you are rinsing, examine the quinoa and pick out kernels that are discolored or any pebbles that may remain. Don't skip this step, the starches in unrinsed quinoa will create an undesirable foamy topping to your bowl.
2. To roast the rinsed quinoa in a saucepan, heat a small pot over medium heat. Once hot, add the rinsed quinoa and allow to toast for three minutes, stirring frequently.
3. Add the non-dairy milk, coconut milk, a pinch of salt, and stir. Bring to a gentle boil over high heat, and then reduce to low and cook, uncovered for twenty to twenty-five minutes. Allow the liquid to simmer; you should see a small amount of bubbling up on the surface, monitor through cooking time, and if it stops simmering, increase the heat to medium-low.
4. Once the quinoa absorbs all the liquid, remove from the heat and add the maple syrup, vanilla, and cocoa powder. Stir thoroughly to combine.

5. Taste and, if needed, adjust the flavor. If the quinoa mixture is too thick, stir in more non-dairy milk, if you would like it sweeter add more maple syrup or sprinkle in coconut sugar. If it's not chocolatey enough, mix in more cocoa powder.

Optional Toppings:
To jazz this dish up, you can add some toppings to each serving.
- Vegan chocolate square
- Sliced banana
- Sliced strawberries
- Blueberries
- Raspberries
- Hemp seeds
- Slivered almonds
- Shredded coconut

Breakfast Twenty-Nine Quinoa & Cinnamon Breakfast Bowl

Nutritional information per serving:

Calories	236	Carbs	40g	Iron	40%
Sugar	4g	Protein	8g	Magnesium	15%
Fiber	4g	Fat	4g		

What You Need:

- Uncooked white quinoa - 1 cup (200g)
- Non-dairy milk - 2 cups (472ml)
- Cinnamon - 1—2 sticks
- Vanilla extract - 1 tsp (5ml)
- Pinch of salt

What to Do:

1. In a fine, mesh strainer, rinse the quinoa for two minutes. As you are rinsing, examine the quinoa and pick out kernels that are discolored or any pebbles that may remain. Don't skip this step, the starches in unrinsed quinoa will create an undesirable foamy topping to your bowl.
2. Roast the rinsed quinoa in a saucepan. Heat a small pot over medium heat. Once hot, add the rinsed quinoa and allow to toast for three minutes, stirring frequently.
3. Add the non-dairy milk, a pinch of salt, and stir. Place the cinnamon sticks upright in the saucepan, as emerged as you can get. Bring to a gentle boil over high heat, and then reduce to low and cook, uncovered for twenty to twenty-five minutes. Allow the liquid to simmer. You should see a small amount of bubbling up on the surface, monitor throughout the cooking time, and if it stops simmering, increase the heat to medium-low.
4. Once all the liquid is absorbed by the quinoa, remove from the heat, pull out the cinnamon sticks.
5. To serve, divide the quinoa among four dishes and finish off with the toppings of your choice. If you want a consistency more like porridge, warm some non-dairy milk (in the microwave or saucepan) and pour over the cooked quinoa, then add your toppings.

Optional Toppings:
- Maple syrup
- Coconut sugar
- Brown sugar
- Nutmeg, cardamom, or garam masala
- Fresh sliced peaches
- Sliced banana
- Mixed berries
- Peanut butter and/or jam
- Slivered almonds
- Granola

Nutritional information per serving:

Calories	141	Carbs	22g	Calcium	40%
Sugar	4g	Protein	3g	Iron	8%
Fiber	3g	Fat	3g		

What You Need:
- Whole wheat flour - 1 cup (200g)
- Baking powder - 1 tbsp (15g)
- Salt - 0.5 tsp (2.5g)
- Non-dairy milk - 1 cup (236ml)
- Olive oil - 2 tbsp (30ml)
- Maple syrup - 2 tbsp (30ml)
- Vanilla extract - 1 tsp (5ml)

What to Do:
1. Whisk together the dry ingredients—flour, baking powder, and salt, in a medium-sized mixing bowl. In a different mixing bowl, mix the wet ingredients—non-dairy milk, olive oil, maple syrup and, vanilla extract. Whisk the wet ingredients thoroughly.
2. Pour the wet ingredients into the dry ingredients bowl and stir until combined. Do not over mix, but do ensure most of the lumps are gone, it's ok if a few small ones remain. If you're adding extras—like blueberries of chocolate chips—do so now and gently fold into the batter. To allow the baking powder to react, let the batter rest for five minutes.
3. While the batter rests, heat a nonstick skillet over medium heat. If you have an electric skillet heat to 350 degrees Fahrenheit (176 degrees Celsius). To test if the surface of the pan is hot, splash a few drops of water on the surface. If the water sizzles on contact, you are ready to cook.
4. It is optional to lightly oil the surface of the pan with cooking spray. It may help with the pancakes not sticking to the pan, and it will depend on your specific tools.

5. Use a 0.25 cup (60ml) measuring tool to scoop the batter onto the warm skillet. Cook for two to three minutes until small bubbles start to form on the surface. Wait until the edges of the pancake are cooked before flipping, they will look matte, and you can easily work a spatula under the entire rim of the pancake. Once flipped, cook for one to two minutes or until it is golden brown.
6. With the rest of the batter, repeat the process above. Monitor the heat and adjust as needed. If the pancakes are sticking, apply, or reapply some oil to the pan in between each pancake.
7. Serve warm with syrup or add on non-dairy butter, coconut whipped cream, fresh berries, honey, or jam.

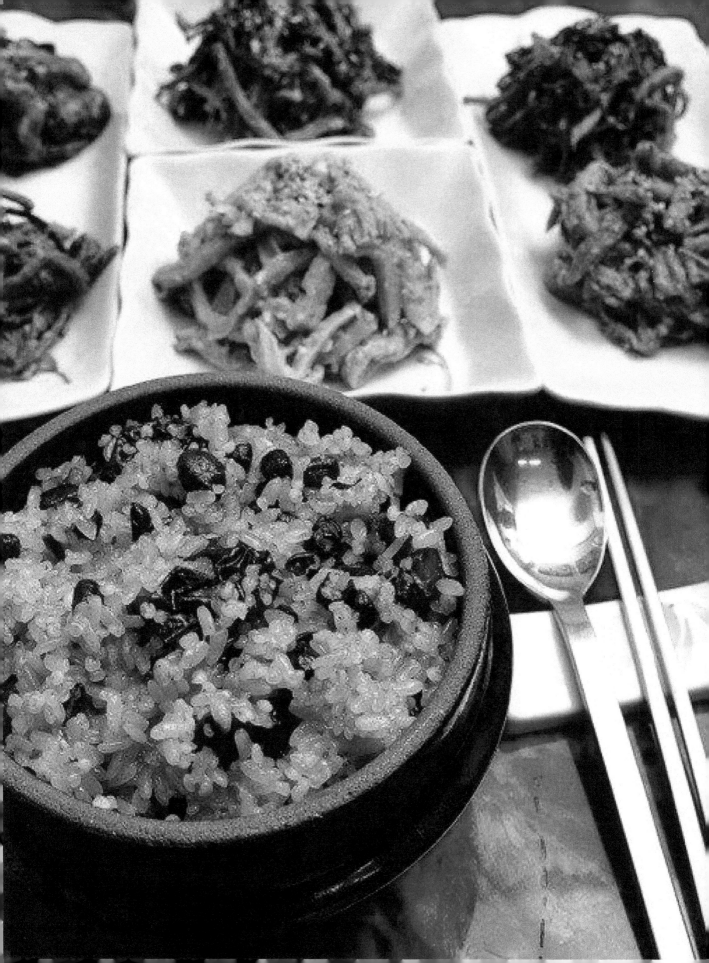

Chapter 8: Lunch Recipes

Lunch One - Caesar Salad

Nutritional Information Per Serving: 500 Calories, 52 grams of Fat, 42 grams of Carbs, 13 grams of Protein

Time: 30 minutes

Serving Size: 4 servings

Ingredients:

- 2 cups sourdough bread, crumbled/cubed
- 2 tablespoons avocado oil
- 4 cups kale
- 2 cups arugula
- 2 avocados, pitted and diced
- ⅓ cup tahini
- 2 lemons, squeezed into juice
- 1 tablespoon apple cider vinegar
- 1 tablespoon olive oil
- 3 cloves garlic, diced
- sea salt and black pepper to preference

Directions:

1. Preheat oven to 350 Fahrenheit or 177 Celsius. Line a baking sheet with parchment paper.
2. Combine the bread, avocado oil, garlic powder, salt and pepper in a bowl. Mix well.
3. Pour the bread onto the baking sheet.
4. Bake for 10 minutes. Remove pan from oven and stir bread.
5. Return the bread to oven for additional 10 minutes.
6. While the bread is cooking mix the arugula, kale, and avocado in a bowl. Place in the refrigerator until the salad is ready to be consumed.

7. In a mason jar or blender, place tahini, lemon juice, apple cider vinegar, olive oil, garlic, salt and pepper. Shake or blend until dressing is smooth. Add water to reach desired consistency.

8. When the croutons are complete, add everything to the salad and serve!

Lunch Two - Buffalo Chickpeas

Nutritional Information Per Serving: 230 Calories, 6 grams of Fat, 34 grams of Carbs, 10 grams of Protein

Time: 10 minutes

Serving Size: 2 servings

Ingredients:

- 1 can chickpeas, drained and rinsed
- 2 tablespoons tahini
- ¼ cup hot sauce
- 1 teaspoon onion powder
- 1 teaspoon smoked paprika
- 1 stalk celery, diced

Directions:

1. Place all ingredients except the celery in a food processor or blender and pulse to reach the desired consistency. You can also place all ingredients in a bowl and mash them together with a fork.
2. Stir in the chopped celery.
3. Serve on bread with fixings or over a salad. This can also be enjoyed plain or with crackers.

Lunch Three - Veg Wrap

Nutritional Information Per Serving: 550 Calories, 18 grams of Fat, 70 grams of Carbs, 18 grams of Protein

Time: 5 minutes

Serving Size: 1 serving

Ingredients:
- ½ cup cooked rice
- 1 whole wheat tortilla
- ½ avocado
- 2 tablespoons hummus (optional)
- ¼ cucumber, sliced
- ½ carrot stalk, sliced
- ½ cup black beans, drained and rinsed

Directions:

1. Prepare the rice and chop vegetables.
2. Place everything in tortilla along with your favorite vegan dressing. The Cesar dressing prepared for *Lunch One* is an excellent option.

Lunch Four- Egg Salad

Nutritional Information Per Serving: 255 Calories, 20 grams of Fat, 8 grams of Carbs, 14 grams of Protein

Time: 10 minutes

Serving Size: 4 servings

Ingredients:
- 1 block tofu, medium firm
- 6 tablespoons vegan mayonnaise
- 2 tablespoons nutritional yeast

- 2 teaspoons yellow mustard
- ¼ teaspoon turmeric
- 1 medium onion, chopped (optional)
- 4 stalks celery (chopped)
- Himalayan salt and black pepper to preference

Directions:
1. Drain and lightly press tofu to remove as much water as possible.
2. Combine all ingredients except onion and celery.
3. Use a spatula to mash everything together.
4. Fold in celery and onion.
5. Serve with bread, crackers, or over salad.

Lunch Five- Lunch Tacos

Nutritional Information Per Serving: 525 Calories, 21 grams of Fat, 70 grams of Carbs, 23 grams of Protein

Time: 5 minutes

Serving Size: 1 serving

Ingredients:

- ¼ cup black beans, drained and rinsed
- ½ avocado, pitted and diced
- ½ cup corn
- 2 tablespoons lime juice
- ⅓ cup cilantro, roughly chopped
- ¼ cup hummus
- 3 small corn tortillas

Directions:

1. Microwave or use a skillet to warm beans, corn, and tortillas.
2. Spread the hummus onto the tortillas evenly.
3. Add the remaining toppings and serve.

Nutritional Information Per Serving: 600 Calories, 27 grams of Fat, 75 grams of Carbs, 19 grams of Protein

Time: 5 minutes

Serving Size: 1 serving

Ingredients:

- 4 cups raw spinach
- ½ cup chickpeas
- 1 cup quinoa, cooked
- ½ avocado
- ½ cup carrots, finely shredded
- 1 small red onion, diced
- 2 tablespoons olive oil
- 2 tablespoons apple cider vinegar
- sea salt and black pepper to preference

Directions:

1. Assemble the bowl by mixing everything together or strategically placing on the sides.
2. Drizzle the olive oil, apple cider vinegar, salt, and pepper over the top. You can also use your favorite vegan dressing if preferred and omit the oil.

Nutritional Information Per Serving: 400 Calories, 21 grams of Fat, 38 grams of Carbs, 14 grams of Protein

Time: 15 minutes

Serving Size: 1 serving

Ingredients:

For the Sandwich:
- ½ cup mushrooms, sliced
- 1 small onion, sliced
- ¼ cup red bell peppers, finely chopped
- 1 teaspoon of olive oil
- 2 pieces of sourdough bread

For the Sauce:
- ¼ cup fresh basil leaves
- ⅔ cup macadamia nuts, raw
- 1 teaspoon garlic powder
- 2 teaspoons nutritional yeast
- ½ tablespoon olive oil
- sea salt and black pepper to preference

Directions:

1. To prepare the sauce, place all ingredients into a food processor. Blend until smooth.
2. For the sandwich, place mushrooms, onion, red bell pepper, and small amount of oil into a skillet. Sauté until soft. This can be done the evening before and warmed up at work if necessary.
3. Toast or heat the bread.
4. Add vegetables and sauce to bread and serve as a sandwich.

Lunch Eight - Pasta Salad

Nutritional Information Per Serving: 305 Calories, 6 grams of Fat, 45 grams of Carbs, 15 grams of Protein

Time: 20 minutes

Serving Size: 3 servings

Ingredients:

For the Salad:

- 5 oz dry pasta
- ½ red bell pepper, chopped
- 1 medium onion, chopped
- 2 small tomatoes, diced
- ¼ cucumber, diced
- ½ cup dill pickles, chopped

Dressing:
- 1½ cups white beans, drained and rinsed
- ¼ cup oat milk
- 2 tablespoons hulled hemp seeds
- 2 teaspoons of garlic powder
- ½ tablespoons lemon juice
- ½ tablespoon apple cider vinegar

Directions:

1. Cook pasta via the instructions on the packaging. Drain when finished.
2. In a blender or food processor add all dressing ingredients and blend until smooth.
3. Add the dressing, noodles, and chopped vegetables into a large bowl and mix well. Refrigerate until cold and serve.

Lunch Nine - Stuffed Sweet Potatoes

Nutritional Information Per Serving: 270 Calories, 12 grams of Fat, 36 grams of Carbs, 6 grams of Protein

Time: 45 minutes

Serving Size: 2 servings

Ingredients:

- 1 large sweet potato
- ½ tablespoon avocado oil
- ¼ cup green bell pepper, chopped
- ¼ cup corn
- ¼ cup quinoa

- ½ cup black beans, drained and rinsed
- ½ tablespoon chili powder
- ¼ teaspoon smoked paprika
- ½ avocado, mashed
- hot sauce (optional)

Directions:

1. Preheat oven to 400 Fahrenheit or 205 Celsius.
2. Place sweet potatoes on baking sheet and bake for 40 minutes. Prick the outside of the sweet potato first.
3. Place avocado oil in a non-stick frying pan and add the rest of the ingredients except the avocado.
4. Sauté vegetables for a few minutes.
5. When sweet potatoes are complete, remove from oven and top with vegetables and avocado. Serve immediately or warm when ready to consume.

Lunch Ten - Stir Fry

Nutritional Information Per Serving: 300 Calories, 21 grams of Fat, 20 grams of Carbs, 10 grams of Protein

Time: 25 minutes

Serving Size: 3 servings

Ingredients:

- 1 small onion, chopped
- 2 teaspoons of garlic powder
- 4 cups broccoli florets
- 1 tablespoon ginger, grated
- 1 cup roasted cashews
- 2-3 tablespoons soy sauce
- 1 tablespoon coconut oil
- 1½ cup quinoa (cooked)

Directions:

1. Follow the instructions on package to cook quinoa. Set quinoa aside when finished.
2. In a skillet sauté the onion and broccoli until soft using a little oil to prevent burning.
3. Add in garlic, ginger, cashews, and soy sauce. Stir.
4. Pour over quinoa and enjoy.

Lunch Eleven - Chicken Salad

Nutritional Information Per Serving: 209 Calories, 9 grams of Fat, 26 grams of Carbs, 9 grams of Protein

Time: 15 minutes

Serving Size: 4 servings

Ingredients:

- ½ cup almonds, halved/chopped
- 15 oz chickpeas, drained and rinsed
- 2 celery stalks, roughly chopped
- ½ cup red grapes, halved
- ¼ cup dried cranberries
- ½ cup vegan mayo (or oil)
- 1 tablespoon apple cider vinegar
- salt and pepper to preference

Directions:

1. In a food processor or blender add in almonds, chickpeas, celery, and spices. Pulse until the desired consistency is reached.
2. Add the mixture to a bowl and fold in grapes, cranberries, vegan mayo, and apple cider vinegar.
3. Serve cold over bread or over a salad.

Nutritional Information Per Serving: 195 Calories, 14 grams of Fat, 13 grams of Carbs, 9 grams of Protein

Time: 35 minutes

Serving Size: 4 servings

Ingredients:

- 1 tablespoon olive oil
- 1 medium onion, chopped
- 2 tablespoons garlic, minced
- 1 tablespoon oregano
- 1 tablespoon dried basil
- 24 oz mushrooms, sliced
- 3 tablespoons soy sauce
- 1 can full-fat coconut milk
- sea salt and pepper to preference

Directions:

1. Add olive oil to a large soup pot and warm over medium heat.
2. Add in onions and all spices. Sauté for four minutes.
3. Add mushrooms and all spices listed.
4. Let everything simmer with the lid on for 10 minutes and stir every so often.
5. Remove the lid and simmer for 10 minutes.
6. Add coconut milk and simmer for an additional 10 minutes.
7. Remove from heat and serve warm.

Lunch Thirteen - Nachos

Nutritional Information Per Serving: 540 Calories, 26 grams of Fat, 66 grams of Carbs, 12 grams of Protein

Time: 5 minutes

Serving Size: 1 serving

Ingredients:

- 30 blue corn tortilla chips (2 servings)
- ½ cup vegetarian refried beans
- ½ avocado, pitted/mashed
- ½ lime, juiced
- 1 teaspoon onion powder
- ¼ cup cilantro
- 1 cup salsa

Directions:

1. In a bowl add lime juice, onion powder, and cilantro to the mashed avocado. This serves as guacamole.
2. Assemble chips on a plate.
3. Warm refried beans and pour over chips.
4. Top the chips with guacamole and salsa.

Lunch Fourteen - Lunchbox

Nutritional Information Per Serving: 700 Calories, 30 grams of Fat, 90 grams of Carbs, 13 grams of Protein

Time: 5 minutes

Serving Size: 1 serving

Ingredients:

- 26 multiseed crackers (2 servings)
- ¼ cup hummus
- ½ cup cucumber, sliced
- ¾ cup green grapes
- 1 banana, sliced
- 1 tablespoon almond butter

Directions:

1. Place all ingredients into separate reusable containers or into a divided container.

Note: This recipe serves as more of a snack box and is great for busy days. This can be eaten throughout the day to keep you full!

Lunch Fifteen - Sushi Spring Rolls

Nutritional Information Per Serving: 285 Calories, 4 grams of Fat, 57 grams of Carbs, 6 grams of Protein

Time: 30 minutes

Serving Size: 4 servings

Ingredients:

For the Rolls:
- ¼ cup sushi rice
- 1 tablespoon rice vinegar
- 4 rice papers
- ½ carrot stalk
- ½ cucumber
- ¼ mango
- ½ avocado
- ½ sheet nori algae
- 1 teaspoon black sesame seeds

For the Sauce:
- ½ avocado
- 1 tablespoon almond milk
- 1 teaspoon garlic
- ½ lemon, juiced
- Himalayan salt and black pepper to taste

Directions:

1. Prepare rice using the instructions on the packaging. After completion add in rice vinegar and set aside to cool.
2. Cut all vegetables and mango into long thin strips.
3. Use scissors to cut the nori algae into 4-inch-long strips.
4. Take one rice paper sheet and dip into water for 15 seconds. Place onto a clean towel.
5. Add all fillings onto one half to make for easier rolling. Start with the rice, and then assemble in random order. Finish with the strips of nori algae.
6. Take the rice paper (the side with no filling) and stretch it over to the filling side. You're essential folding the rice paper in half. Fold in the sides and roll until every angle of the rice paper is sealed.
7. Cut the rolls in half to resemble sushi or eat them how they are.
8. Finish by preparing the sauce. Add all the sauce ingredients into a blender and pulse until a smooth consistency appears.

Lunch Sixteen - Barbeque Chickpea Salad with Ranch

Nutritional Information Per Serving: 300 Calories, 8 grams of Fat, 50 grams of Carbs, 13 grams of Protein

Time: 20 minutes

Serving Size: 2 servings

Ingredients:

For the Chickpeas:
- 1½ cup chickpeas, drained and rinsed
- ¼ cup bbq sauce (vegan)

For the Dressing:
- 2 tablespoons tahini
- 2 tablespoons lemon juice
- ½ teaspoon garlic powder
- ½ teaspoon onion powder

- ½ teaspoon apple cider vinegar
- 1 tablespoon water

For the Salad:
- 4 cups arugula
- 1 small red onion, roughly chopped
- ¼ cup corn

Directions:

1. In a medium-sized pan, cook chickpeas and bbq sauce over medium heat. Cook for five to ten minutes or until the sauce starts to get sticky. Stir frequently to prevent burning.
2. In a blender, a food processor, or glass mason jar, add all dressing ingredients. Shake or blend until ingredients are well mixed.
3. Assemble salad by placing ingredients into a large bowl. Add in chickpeas and dressing.
4. Enjoy immediately or store in an airtight container in the refrigerator.

Lunch Seventeen - Meatball Bomber

Nutritional Information Per Meatball: 55 Calories, 3 grams of Fat, 8 grams of Carbs, 4 grams of Protein

Time: 30 minutes

Serving Size: 13 meatballs

Ingredients:

- 1½ cups canned kidney beans, drained and rinsed
- 2 tablespoons garlic, minced
- 1 small red onion, chopped
- 1 teaspoon oregano
- 1 teaspoon soy sauce
- 1 tablespoon tomato paste
- ½ cup rolled oats

- ½ cup mushrooms, chopped
- ⅓ cup sunflower seeds
- sea salt and pepper to preference

Directions:

1. Preheat oven to 350 Fahrenheit or 177 Celsius. Line a baking sheet with parchment paper.
2. Place kidney beans into a large bowl and mash using a fork.
3. In a non-stick frying pan, sauté onions, garlic, and mushrooms until vegetables are soft. Use a dab of oil if necessary. Remove from heat when completed.
4. Add all spices, tomato paste, soy sauce, sautéed vegetables, and oats to the bowl containing the kidney beans. Mix well.
5. Add sunflower seeds to a high-speed blender or food processor and blend until a fine flour-like substance appears. Add it to the bowl containing the other ingredients.
6. Form 13 vegan meatballs and place on a lined baking sheet.
7. Bake for 15 minutes and remove from oven to cool when completed.

Note: These meatballs are excellent alone with marinara sauce or in between bread. Vegan cheese is also available at supermarkets if desired.

Lunch Eighteen - Tomato Soup

Nutritional Information Per Serving: 270 Calories, 22 grams of Fat, 15 grams of Carbs, 3 grams of Protein

Time: 25 minutes

Serving Size: 6 servings

Ingredients:

- 1 tablespoon olive oil
- 1 cup onion, diced
- 2 tablespoons garlic, minced

- 2 tablespoons vegan pesto (See *Lunch 7* for recipe)
- 1 teaspoon oregano
- 28 oz fire roasted tomatoes
- 14.5 oz vegetable broth
- 13.5 oz can coconut milk
- sea salt and black pepper to preference

Directions:

1. In a large pot, heat oil, onion, garlic, salt, and pepper for 5 minutes on medium heat. Stir frequently.
2. Stir in pesto, oregano, tomatoes, and vegetable broth.
3. Turn heat to high and bring to a boil.
4. Lower heat to low and let the soup simmer for 10 minutes. Sir a few times throughout.
5. Transfer the soup to a blender and process until the soup has a smooth consistency.
6. Put the soup back into the pot and add coconut milk.
7. Cook for an additional 5 minutes on low heat before serving and storing.

Lunch Nineteen - Caprese Mozzarella Recipe

Nutritional Information Per Serving: 310 Calories, 8 grams of Fat, 3 grams of Carbs, 10 grams of Protein

Time: 10 minutes (overnight recipe)

Serving Size: 4 servings

Ingredients:

- 14 oz tofu, extra firm
- 1 cup extra virgin olive oil
- 2 tablespoons Italian seasoning
- 1 teaspoon garlic, minced
- sea salt and pepper to preference

Directions:

1. Drain and slice tofu into thin slices. The thinner the better.
2. In a glass container, mix olive oil, garlic, and seasonings.
3. Place the tofu into the mixture and marinate the tofu overnight.
4. The following day you can shred or leave the tofu slices.
5. Serve the tofu cheese over a salad with tomatoes, pesto sauce, or other toppings of choice.

Lunch Twenty - Avocado Toast

Nutritional Information Per Serving: 470 Calories, 50 grams of Fat, 24 grams of Carbs, 8 grams of Protein

Time: 10 minutes

Serving Size: 1 serving

Ingredients:

- 1 slice of vegan bread (see bread recipe, *breakfast 9*)
- ½ avocado, mashed
- ½ medium tomato, sliced
- 2 tablespoons olive oil
- 1 teaspoon garlic powder
- sea salt and black pepper to preference

Directions:

1. Prepare the toast or bread by heating or placing it in the toaster.
2. Prepare the toppings by mashing the avocado and slicing the tomato.
3. Place the avocado and tomato on the toast. Sprinkle the rest of the ingredients to preference.

Lunch Twenty-One - Taco Meat

Nutritional Information Per Serving: 106 Calories, 22 grams of Fat, 10 grams of Carbs, 5 grams of Protein

Time: 15 minutes

Serving Size: 6 servings

Ingredients:

- 1 tablespoon olive oil
- ¼ red onion, roughly chopped
- 2½ cups cooked lentils
- 2 tablespoons taco seasoning (vegan)
- ¼ cup water
- 2 tablespoons hot sauce (optional)
- Himalayan salt and pepper to preference

Directions:

1. In a skillet, add olive oil and onions and sauté over medium heat for two minutes.
2. Add lentils, taco seasoning, hot sauce, and water to the pan and set the heat to low.
3. Let everything simmer for 5 minutes, stirring occasionally.
4. Remove from heat and serve over a salad, protein bowl, taco, or burrito.

Lunch Twenty-Two - Creamy Cauliflower Soup

Nutritional Information Per Serving: 205 Calories, 6 grams of Fat, 30 grams of Carbs, 10 grams of Protein

Time: 45 minutes

Serving Size: 6 servings

Ingredients:

- 1 tablespoon olive oil
- 2 cups leeks, sliced
- 3 garlic cloves, minced
- 6 cups cauliflower, chopped
- ¾ teaspoon nutmeg
- ½ teaspoon of red pepper flakes
- 15 oz can white beans, drained and rinsed
- 4 cups vegetable broth
- 2 cups water
- ¼ cup cashews
- ½ cup nutritional yeast
- sea salt and black pepper to preference

Directions:

1. In a large soup pot, heat oil, leeks, and garlic for two minutes over medium heat.
2. Add in cauliflower and all spices. Allow this to simmer for five minutes.
3. Add beans, vegetable broth, and water. Bring to a boil.
4. Reduce heat and cover. Let the soup cook for 30 minutes on medium-low heat, stirring occasionally.
5. Transfer soup to a blender and add cashews. Puree until the soup is smooth and creamy.
6. Transfer soup back to pot and add nutritional yeast. Stir.
7. Serve with your favorite bread or pumpkin seeds to garnish.

Lunch Twenty-Three - Power Bowl

Nutritional Information Per Serving: 375 Calories, 11 grams of Fat, 35 grams of Carbs, 14 grams of Protein

Time: 5 minutes

Serving Size: 2 servings

Ingredients:

- 1 cup quinoa, cooked
- ½ cup black beans, drained and rinsed
- 10 kalamata olives
- 1 serving caprese mozzarella (see *Lunch 19*)
- ½ cup cucumber, sliced
- 1 cup spinach leaves

Directions:

1. Place all ingredients into a glass container. Assemble by mixing together or by keeping ingredients separate.
2. This lunch can be served hot or cold, and choose your favorite vegan dressing to top if you desire.

Lunch Twenty-Four - Mediterranean Sandwich

Nutritional Information Per Serving: 410 Calories, 28 grams of Fat, 31 grams of Carbs, 10 grams of Protein

Time: 10 minutes

Serving Size: 1 serving

Ingredients:

- ½ cup chickpeas, drained and rinsed
- ½ avocado
- 1 teaspoon lime juice
- ¼ cup red onion, roughly chopped
- small handful of cilantro
- 1 teaspoon garlic powder
- 1 tablespoon olive oil
- 2-3 slices of tomato
- sea salt and pepper to preference

Directions:

1. To make the filling of the sandwich, place chickpeas, avocado, lime juice, red onion, cilantro, garlic powder, salt, and pepper into a small bowl.
2. Use a fork to mash everything together.
3. Take two slices of your favorite, hearty bread and spread the mixture onto the bread. This can be an open- or closed-face sandwich.
4. Add tomato, drizzle olive oil, and enjoy.

Note: Nutrition facts do not include bread.

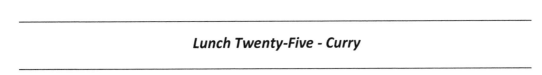

Lunch Twenty-Five - Curry

Nutritional Information Per Serving: 290 Calories, 21 grams of Fat, 23 grams of Carbs, 6 grams of Protein

Time: 25 minutes

Serving Size: 4 servings

Ingredients:

- 1 tablespoon garlic, minced
- 1 medium onion, chopped
- 1 tablespoon tomato paste
- 5 medium tomatoes, chopped
- 14 oz potatoes, cubed
- 14 oz canned coconut milk
- 1 tablespoon curry powder
- 1 teaspoon turmeric
- 1 teaspoon garam masala
- 1 cup spinach
- Himalayan salt and pepper to preference

Directions:

1. In a non-stick saucepan add onion and garlic. Sauté over medium heat for three minutes.

2. Add tomato paste, stir, and simmer for one minute.
3. Add tomatoes and simmer for three minutes. Stir occasionally.
4. Add potatoes, coconut milk, curry, turmeric, and garam masala. Cover and simmer on medium heat for 15 minutes or until potatoes are tender.
5. Stir in spinach and serve.

Note: This recipe is best served with rice, quinoa, or lentils.

Lunch Twenty-Six - Crispy Tofu

Nutritional information per serving:

Calories	95	Carbs	2g	Iron	25%
Sugar	0g	Protein	12g	Calcium	25%
Fiber	1g	Fat	6g		

What You Need:

- Extra Firm Tofu - 14 oz (396g)
- Tamari (soy sauce or coconut amino works too) - 1 tbsp (15ml)
- Nutritional Yeast - 2 tbsp (30g)

Optional Seasoning:
- Garlic powder
- Smoked paprika
- Ground cumin
- Ground ginger
- Black pepper
- Chinese 5 spice
- Toasted sesame seeds

What to Do:

- Ensure your oven is preheated to 425 degrees Fahrenheit (250 degrees Celsius). Open to tofu and drain the excess water. Press the tofu by wrapping it in an absorbent towel and resting something heavy on top—a cookbook or cast-iron skillet. Let it rest for ten to 15 minutes.

- Once the tofu is pressed and as dry as you can get it, cut the block into bite-sized cubes.
- Add the cubed and pressed tofu to a large bowl. Pour the tamari over the tofu and use a large spoon or spatula to gently coat each cube of tofu with the tamari, being careful not to break up the cubes. Add the nutritional yeast (plus any optional seasonings you wish) and toss the bowl to allow the flakes to coat each cube, use the spoon or spatula to gently flip, and ensure every cube of tofu is covered with nutritional yeast. Add more as necessary.
- Line a medium-sized baking sheet with parchment paper and transfer the tofu cubes to the baking sheet. Arrange in single rows with enough space between each piece, so they are not touching.
- Bake in the oven for twenty minutes, then remove and flip each cube over. Return to the oven and bake for another twenty minutes or until the tofu cubes are crispy and golden.
- Allow the cubes to cool and store in the fridge for up to one week. Add to your favorite salad or soup recipe from below.

Lunch Twenty-Seven Thai Noodle Salad

Nutritional information per serving:

Calories	286	Carbs	40g	Sodium	6%
Sugar	13g	Protein	4g	Iron	2%
Fiber	3g	Fat	13g		

What You Need:

- Soba noodles - 6 oz (170g)
- Shredded veggies - 4 cups (800g). A mix of red cabbage, carrots and radish
- Red pepper - 1, large, sliced into thin strips

- Green onion - 3, sliced for topping
- Fresh cilantro (or basil or mint) - 0.5 cup (100g), chopped
- Jalapeno, minced - 1 tbsp (15g)
- Crushed peanuts - 0.25 cup (50g), roasted

Peanut Thai Sauce (make a double batch and save for another meal. It's that good)
- Ginger - 3 thin slices, roughly the size of a quarter each
- Garlic - 1 large clove, minced
- Peanut butter - 0.25 cup (50g)
- Orange juice - 0.5 of an orange, squeezed
- Lime juice - 1 lime, squeezed
- Soy sauce - 2 tbsp (30ml) Coconut aminos works too, tamari is too dark
- Agave syrup - 3 tbsp (45ml)
- Toasted sesame oil - 3 tbsp (45ml)
- Cayenne pepper (or hot sauce) - 0.25 tsp (1.25g)
- Pinch of salt

What to Do:
1. Cook the noodles according to the orders on the package. When cooked, drain and run under cool running water to chill and stop the cooking process.
2. While the pasta cooks, prepare the Thai peanut sauce. Add all the sauce ingredients to a blender and run until smooth.
3. In a large serving bowl, place the shredded veggies, bell pepper, green onions, cilantro (or basil or mint), and jalapeno and toss everything together. Add to chilled noodles to the bowl and toss again to mix everything thoroughly.
4. Pour the peanut sauce over the bowl and mix well

*If you made a double batch pour out half into a sealable container before adding to the salad.

Toss everything together to combine. Taste and adjust as desired. Add more heat with hot sauce of more jalapenos, make a little sweeter by adding in a small amount of the agave syrup or squeeze more lime to make the dish a bit more tart. Garnish with roasted peanuts, cilantro (or basil or mint), and a lime wedge.

Nutritional information per serving:

Calories	332	Carbs	51g	Potassium	28%
Sugar	6g	Protein	16g	Iron	28%
Fiber	17g	Fat	7g		

What You Need:

Black Beans
- Black beans - 1 15oz can (425g), drained and rinsed
- Chili powder - 2 tsp (10g)
- Cumin - 1 tsp (5g)
- Garlic powder - 1 tsp (5g)
- Smoked paprika - 1 tsp (5g)
- Cayenne - 1 tsp (5g)
- Salt - 1 tsp (5g)
- Water - 0.25 cup (50ml)

Crispy Chickpeas
- Chickpeas - 1 15 oz (425g) can, rinsed and drained
- Chili powder - 1 tsp (5g)
- Cumin - 1 tsp (5g)
- Salt - 1 tsp (5g)
- Cinnamon - 1 tsp (5g)

Salad
- Green leaf or romaine lettuce - 1 head, chopped
- Tomatoes - 1-2, medium, diced
- Red pepper - 1, large, diced
- Avocado - 1, large, diced
- Fresh corn kernels (or frozen, cooked and chilled) - 1 cup (ml)

Vegan Southwest Creamy Ranch Dressing

Double the recipe, save it in the fridge and put this on everything, and I do mean everything)

- Water - 0.5 cup
- Cashews - 0.75 cup (150g). Soaked for 2 hours
- Lemon juice - 1 lemon, squeezed
- Apple cider vinegar - 1 tbsp (30ml)
- Garlic - 1 clove
- Cumin - 1 tsp (5g)
- Dried dill - 1 tsp (5g)
- Chives - 1 tsp (5g), minced
- Onion powder - 1 tsp (5g)
- Smoked paprika - 1 tsp (5g)
- Dried oregano - 1 tsp (5g)
- Salt - 0.50 tsp (2g)

What to Do:

For the Dressing:
1. In a blend with a high-speed setting, place all the ingredients and run until smooth. Add more water by the tablespoon as needed to get the consistency you desire.

For the Salad:
1. Ensure your oven is preheated to 400 degrees Fahrenheit.
2. In a medium bowl, toss the drained and rinsed chickpeas with the spices (chili powder, cumin, salt, cinnamon).
3. Place the seasoned chickpeas on a medium-sized baking sheet lined with parchment paper in one even layer, with room between each chickpea — Bake for twenty to thirty minutes. At the ten to fifteen-minute mark, remove chickpeas from the oven and shake them around on the baking sheet. Return the chickpeas to the oven and continue to bake until slightly crunchy. Remove from the oven, and they will continue to get crispy as they cool.
4. While the chickpeas bake, prepare the black beans. In a medium bowl, toss the drained and rinsed black beans with the spices (chili powder, cumin, garlic powder, smoked paprika, cayenne, salt). Over medium heat, warm a frying pan, and add the spice coated beans to the pan with 0.75 cup of water. Stir occasionally as the beans warm for five to six minutes.

5. Assemble to salad ingredients. Toss together the lettuce, tomatoes, pepper, avocado, and corn in a large serving bowl. Plate the lettuce mixture into individual servings and add the black beans to each dish. Top with the crispy chickpeas and drizzle each serving with the creamy ranch dressing.

Lunch Twenty-Nine - Curried Tofu Salad

Nutritional information per serving:

Calories	215	Carbs	21g	Iron	25%
Sugar	13g	Protein	7g	Potassium	15%
Fiber	3g	Fat	13g		

What You Need:

- Extra firm tofu - 8 oz (226g). Cut into small half inch cubes
- Olive oil - 1 tbsp (15ml)
- Salt, and pepper - 0.5 tsp (2.5g)
- Cashews - 0.25 cup (50g), chopped
- Golden raisins - 0.25 cup (50g)
- Red onion (or green onion) - 0.25 cup (50g), diced
- Cilantro - 0.25 cup (50g), chopped
- Celery - 0.25 cup (50g), diced
- Apple - 0.25 cup (50g), diced
- Cayenne (optional) - 0.5 tsp (2.5g)
- Curry powder - 3 tbsp (45g)
- Vegan mayo - 3 tbsp (45ml)
- Agave (or maple syrup) - 1 tbsp (15ml)
- Apple cider vinegar - 1 tbsp (15ml)

What to Do:

1. Press the tofu by wrapping it in an absorbent towel and resting something heavy, like a cookbook or cast-iron skillet, on top of the tofu. Let rest for ten

to fifteen minutes. Once the excess water has been drained, cut the tofu into small cubes, blot with the absorbent towel again to soak up the last of the excess water.

2. Warm a large skillet over medium heat, add the olive oil, salt and pepper, and tofu cubes. Brown the tofu as best you can on all sides. Stir and flip as the tofu cooks to allow each side of the cubes the opportunity to turn golden. Once most sides are cooked, remove from heat and place in a medium-sized serving bowl.

3. Add the cashews, raisins, onions, cilantro, celery, and apples and stir gently.

4. Add the curry powder, cayenne, vegan mayo, agave, and vinegar and stir to mix everything thoroughly.

5. Taste and adjust seasoning as you wish, with more salt, pepper or heat with more cayenne or curry powder.

6. Serve as-is in a bowl or make it more heart in a wrap or pita bread, add some spinach to keep the tortilla or pita from getting soggy. To keep the carbs lower, serve over a bed of mixed salad greens and top with sprouts and half a diced avocado.

Lunch Thirty Middle Eastern Chickpea Salad

Nutritional information per serving:

Calories	260	Carbs	40g	Iron	19%
Sugar	4g	Protein	16g	Potassium	10%
Fiber	10g	Fat	4g		

What You Need:

- Garbanzo beans (aka Chickpeas) - 2 15 oz (850g) cans, drained and rinsed
- Red pepper - 1, large, diced
- Yellow pepper - 1, large, diced
- Tomatoes - 1 cup, diced
- Cucumber - 1, large, diced
- Green onions - 5, diced

- Fresh mint - 1 cup (200g), chopped
- Fresh parsley - 1 cup (200g), chopped
- Garlic - 1 clove, minced
- Olive oil - 0.5 cup (118ml)
- Lemon juice - 1 lemon, squeezed
- Lemon Zest - 0.5 lemon peel, grated
- Sumac (optional) - 1 tsp (5g)
- Cayenne (optional) - 0.25 tsp (2.5g)

Optional Serving Choices:

Pita bread, tortilla wrap, mixed salad greens, sprouts, avocado, hummus, or tahini sauce

What to Do:

1. In a large serving bowl, place the chickpeas, chopped vegetables, and herbs.
2. Add the spices if you're using them and drizzle with olive oil and lemon juice. Stir thoroughly to combine all ingredients well.
3. Serve as-is in a bowl and top with any options listed above or place in a slice of pita bread or tortilla wrap. If using a pita or wrap, set some fresh spinach between bread and salad to prevent it from getting soggy.

Lunch Thirty-One - Crunchy Veggie Wrap with Apples and Spicy Hummus

---

Nutritional information per serving:

Calories	121	Carbs	27g	Sodium	10%
Sugar	9g	Protein	4g	Potassium	5%
Fiber	6g	Fat	2g		

What You Need:

- Spicy hummus (or any sandwich spread) - 4 tbsp (60ml)
- Dairy-free yogurt, unsweetened - 2 tbsp (30ml)

- Lemon juice - 0.5 lemon, squeezed
- Broccoli slaw (purchased) - 0.5 cup (100g)
- Apple - 0.25, sliced thin
- Lettuce (romaine, green leaf or spinach) - 1 cup (200g)
- Flour or corn tortilla - 1

What to Do:

1. In a small bowl, mix yogurt and lemon juice and add the broccoli slaw, stir to combine.
2. Assemble the wrap by spreading the spicy hummus onto the whole tortilla, place the lettuce on top of the hummus. Pile the broccoli slaw over the lettuce on one half of the tortilla and top with the sliced apple. Fold the edges of the tortilla in and then roll tightly from the end with the slaw.

Lunch Thirty-Two - VBLT—Vegan-Bacon Lettuce and Tomato Sandwich

---

Nutritional information per serving:

Calories	272	Carbs	32g	Iron	14%
Sugar	6g	Protein	19g	Calcium	6%
Fiber	5g	Fat	10g		

What You Need:

- Maple smoked tempeh - 8 oz (226g)
- Lettuce leaves (romaine or green leaf) - 1 cup (200g)
- Tomato - 1 large, sliced
- Vegan mayo - 0.25 cup (50ml)
- Olive oil - 1 tsp (5ml)
- Whole grain bread - 4 slices, lightly toasted
- Vegan butter - 1 tbsp (15ml)

Optional—1 avocado, sliced or mashed in with the vegan mayo and two slices of vegan cheese

What to Do:

1. Warm a skillet over medium heat and add the olive oil. Once heated, add tempeh and cook on both sides until lightly crisped.
2. While the tempeh cooks toast the bread, lightly butter each piece then layer on vegan mayo.
3. Add the cooked tempeh, if using a vegan cheese add on top of the warm tempeh, then add the lettuce and tomato.
4. Enjoy as-is or with one of the soups listed below.

Lunch Thirty-Three - Chickpea Noodle Soup

Nutritional information per serving:

Calories	260	Carbs	44g	Vitamin A	210%
Sugar	7g	Protein	7g	Calcium	15%
Fiber	4g	Fat	5g	Micro c	

What You Need:

- Olive oil - 2 tbsp (30ml)
- Garlic - 4 cloves, minced
- Onion - 2, small, chopped
- Carrots - 4, peeled and sliced into thin discs
- Celery - 4 stocks, sliced thin
- Dried thyme - 2 tbsp (30g)
- Dried sage - 1 tbsp (15g)
- Bay leaf - 1
- Vegetable broth - 8 cups (1,888ml)
- Rotini noodles - 8 oz (226g). Any shape of short noodles will work
- Chickpeas - 1 15 oz (425g) can drained and rinsed

What to Do:

1. Heat the olive oil over medium heat in a large soup pot. Add the onions, carrots, and celery and cook for five minutes until softened. Add the garlic, thyme, and sage, stir to combine and cook for two minutes.

2. Add the vegetable broth, stirring to scrape the bottom of the soup pot, bringing up any charred-on spices. Add the bay leaf and bring the broth to a boil.

3. Once boiling, add the noodles and chickpeas and cook for eight to ten minutes until the noodles are al dente. Remove from heat and taste, add salt and pepper to your liking.

Lunch Thirty-Four - Mexican Lentil Soup

Nutritional information per serving:

Calories	235	Carbs	32g	Iron	15%
Sugar	13g	Protein	9g	Potassium	10%
Fiber	10g	Fat	7g		

What You Need:

- Olive oil - 2 tbsp (30ml)
- Onion - 1 medium, diced
- Carrots - 3, peeled and diced
- Celery - 3 stocks—diced
- Red pepper - 1, large, diced
- Garlic - 5 cloves, minced
- Cumin - 2 tbsp (30g)
- Smoked paprika - 1 tsp (5g)
- Oregano= 1 tsp (5g)
- Ancho chili powder - 1 tsp (5g)
- Diced tomatoes - 1 15oz (425g) can

- Diced green chilies - 2 4oz (226g) cans
- Green lentils - 2 cups (400g), rinsed and sorted
- Vegetable broth - 8 cups (1,888ml)
- Salt to taste

Optional Toppings:
- Dash of hot sauce
- Avocado - 1, large
- non-dairy sour cream - 2 tbsp (30ml)
- Fresh cilantro
- Toasted flatbread

What to Do:

1. Heat the olive oil over medium heat in a large soup pot. Add onion, carrots, and celery and sauté for five minutes until they begin to soften. Add the garlic and bell pepper and sauté for three minutes. Add the cumin, smoked paprika, oregano, and ancho chili powder, sauté for one minute, stirring constantly.

2. Add tomatoes, chilis, lentils, broth, and salt. Reduce the heat to a medium/low if needed and allow it to simmer. Place the lid on the pot, tilted so some steam can get out. Simmer the soup for thirty to forty minutes, until the lentils are tender. Season to taste with salt and pepper and serve with any, or all, of the optional toppings.

Chapter 9: Dinner Recipes

Dinner One - Broccoli Cheese Dish

Nutritional Information Per Serving: 380 Calories, 9 grams of Fat, 65 grams of Carbs, 10 grams of Protein

Time: 45 minutes

Serving Size: 6 servings

Ingredients:

- 2 cups brown rice, dry
- 1 teaspoon avocado oil
- 2 heads of broccoli, roughly chopped
- 1 medium onion, chopped
- 2 large tomatoes, peeled and cubed
- ½ cup carrots, chopped
- 2 cups water
- ⅔ cup cashews
- 1 tablespoon garlic, minced
- 2 tablespoons nutritional yeast
- sea salt and black pepper to preference

Directions:

1. In a large non-stick saucepan, cook rice using the directions on the packaging. When the rice is finished, set the rice into a large bowl to cool.
2. In the same pan used before, add olive oil and broccoli. Cook for two minutes over medium heat.
3. Add two tablespoons of water to the pan and steam broccoli for five minutes or until tender.
4. Remove broccoli when finished and set aside.
5. In the saucepan, add onion, potatoes, carrots, and 2 inches of water. Cover and bring water to a boil.
6. Reduce heat and simmer for 15 minutes or until vegetables are soft.

7. Add onions, potatoes and carrots to a blender.
8. Add 1 cup of water, cashews, spices, and nutritional yeast to the blender. Blend until smooth.
9. Add the broccoli and rice back to the saucepan. Cover with the sauce from the blender and stir.
10.   Enjoy warm.

Dinner Two - Mushroom Stew

Nutritional Information Per Serving: 370 Calories, 13 grams of Fat, 48 grams of Carbs, 8 grams of Protein

Time: 1 hour 30 minutes (15 mins prep)

Serving Size: 2 servings

Ingredients:

For the Stew:
- 2 tablespoons olive oil
- 1 onion, chopped
- 1 tablespoon garlic, minced
- 2 cups vegetable broth
- 2 tablespoons flour
- 1 carrot, diced
- 1 large potato, cubed
- 2 cups mushrooms, stems removed
- ½ cup peas
- 1 tablespoon tomato paste
- 1 cup red wine
- Himalayan salt and black pepper to preference

Directions:

1. In a large pot, add 1 tablespoon olive oil, onions, and garlic. Simmer over medium heat for 10 minutes.

2. In a smaller pot, add 1 tablespoon of olive oil and flour over medium-low heat. Whisk until no lumps remain and slowly add in vegetable broth. Whisk until smooth.
3. Add carrots, potatoes, mushrooms, peas, tomato paste, salt, and pepper to the pot containing the onions/garlic. Stir.
4. Add red wine into the large pot containing the vegetables. Simmer on medium heat for three minutes.
5. Combine the small pot ingredients into the large stew pot. Stir.
6. Cover the pot and simmer on low heat for one hour.
7. Remove from heat, enjoy, and store any leftovers in the refrigerator.

Note: This recipe is best served over mashed potatoes, rice, or quinoa.

Dinner Three - Baked Ziti

Nutritional Information Per Serving: 376 Calories, 10 grams of Fat, 51 grams of Carbs, 15 grams of Protein

Time: 50 minutes

Serving Size: 4 servings

Ingredients:

For the Cheese:
- ¾ cups cashews, raw
- ¼ cup water
- 2 tablespoons lemon juice
- 2 tablespoons nutritional yeast
- 1 teaspoon garlic, minced
- ¼ teaspoon onion powder
- Himalayan salt and pepper to preference

The Ziti:
- ½ pound ziti noodles (vegan)
- 1 jar marinara sauce (12.5 ounces)
- ½ bag vegan shredded cheese

Directions:

1. Preheat oven to 375 degrees or 190 degrees Celsius. Grease a nine-by-thirteen casserole dish.
2. Soak the cashews in boiling hot water for five minutes. Drain and place in blender when finished.
3. Add water, lemon juice, nutritional yeast, garlic, onion powder, salt, and pepper to the blender.
4. Blend until smooth and creamy.
5. Prepare the pasta using the directions on the package.
6. When the noodles are finished, pour them into the casserole dish.
7. Pour marinara sauce over the noodles and stir.
8. Sprinkle vegan cheese over the top.
9. Place dish into oven and bake uncovered for 25 minutes.

Dinner Four - Vegan Chili

Nutritional Information Per Serving: 390 Calories, 8 grams of Fat, 55 grams of Carbs, 28 grams of Protein

Time: 40 minutes

Serving Size: 64 servings

Ingredients:

- 14 ounces taco meat (see recipe from *Lunch 21*)
- 1 medium onion, diced
- 2 tablespoon garlic, minced
- 2 28-oz cans crushed tomatoes
- 2 15-oz cans black beans, drained and rinsed
- 1 15-oz can kidney beans, drained and rinsed
- 1 cup water
- 3 tablespoons chili powder
- 1 teaspoon smoked paprika
- ¼ teaspoon cayenne pepper
- 1 tablespoon cocoa powder
- sea salt and pepper to preference

Directions:

1. Prepare taco meat using recipe from *Lunch 21*.
2. In a large pot, add a few tablespoons of water, onion, and garlic. Simmer over medium heat for five minutes.
3. Add all other chili ingredients excluding the taco meat. Stir.
4. Bring to a boil and then lower heat to low.
5. Simmer for 20 minutes and stir occasionally.
6. Stir in taco meat.
7. Serve with tortilla chips, hot sauce, chives, tomatoes, avocado or any other desired toppings.

Dinner Five - Alfredo Sauce Recipe

Nutritional Information Per Serving: 435 Calories, 19 grams of Fat, 50 grams of Carbs, 16 grams of Protein

Time: 15 minutes

Serving Size: 3 servings

Ingredients:

- ¾ cups cashews, raw
- 1 tablespoon olive oil
- ½ medium sized onion
- 1 teaspoon garlic, minced
- 1 cup cashew milk
- 4 tablespoons nutritional yeast
- ½ tablespoon lemon juice
- Himalayan salt and pepper to preference

Directions:

1. Boil 2 cups of water and pour over cashews in a glass bowl. Allow them to soak for five minutes.
2. In a skillet, add oil, onion, and garlic. Sauté for five minutes.
3. Drain the cashews and place in a high-speed blender.

4. Add the onions, garlic, cashew milk, nutritional yeast, lemon juice, salt, and pepper. Blend until smooth.
5. Return sauce to the pan to warm, or store until you're ready to consume.

Note: This recipe makes a great addition to pastas, potatoes, and other dishes.

Dinner Six - Fajitas

Nutritional Information Per Serving: 120 Calories, 5 grams of Fat, 12 grams of Carbs, 3 grams of Protein

Time: 35 minutes

Serving Size: 3 servings

Ingredients:

- 2 cups cauliflower, in florets
- 1 red pepper, sliced
- 1 green pepper, sliced
- 1 small onion, sliced
- 3 tablespoons olive oil
- ½ tablespoon chili powder
- ½ teaspoon cumin
- ½ teaspoon onion powder
- sea salt and pepper to preference

Directions:

1. Preheat oven to 425 Fahrenheit or 218 Celsius. Line a sheet pan with parchment paper.
2. In a large bowl, mix all spices together.
3. Toss in all vegetables and olive oil. Mix well to evenly coat the vegetables.
4. Add the mixture to a sheet pan and roast for 25 minutes or until vegetables have crispy edges.
5. Serve with tortillas or over a salad. Serve with toppings like guacamole, hot sauce, and rice if preferred.

Nutritional Information Per Serving: 305 Calories, 17 grams of Fat, 28 grams of Carbs, 10 grams of Protein

Time: 1 hour

Serving Size: 4 servings

Ingredients:

- ½ tablespoon olive oil
- 1 small onion, roughly chopped
- 4 ounces of mushrooms, finely chopped
- 1 small carrot, peeled and diced
- ¾ cup walnuts
- 1 cup cooked lentils
- 1 tablespoon ground flaxseed
- 1 tablespoon ketchup
- 1 tablespoon Worcestershire sauce
- ¼ cup breadcrumbs
- sea salt and pepper to preference

Directions:

1. Preheat oven to 350 Fahrenheit or 177 Celsius. Line a standard loaf pan with parchment paper.
2. Add olive oil, onions, mushrooms, and carrots to a large pan.
3. Sauté on medium heat for five minutes. After, set aside.
4. Add walnuts to a food processor and pulse a few times. Add in lentils and pulse a few more times.
5. In a large bowl, add the lentils, walnuts, vegetables, flaxseed, ketchup, Worcestershire sauce, salt, and pepper. Mix well.
6. Fold in breadcrumbs.
7. Transfer mixture to loaf pan and press the mixture to even. Cover with foil.
8. Bake for 30 minutes.
9. Remove from oven and serve warm. Add additional ketchup if desired.

Nutritional Information Per Burger: 220 Calories, 6 grams of Fat, 30 grams of Carbs, 9 grams of Protein

Time: 45 minutes

Serving Size: 12 burgers

Ingredients:

- ¼ cup ground flax
- ½ cup water
- 3 cups black beans, drained and rinsed
- 1 cup cashews
- 1½ cup rice
- ½ cup parsley
- 1½ cup shredded carrots
- ⅓ cup green onions, chopped
- 1 cup breadcrumbs
- 2 tablespoons chili powder
- 1 tablespoon garlic, minced
- 1 teaspoon sea salt

Directions:

1. Preheat oven to 350 Fahrenheit or 177 Celsius. Line two baking sheets with parchment paper.
2. In a cup, add flaxseed and water. Put in refrigerator.
3. In a large bowl add black beans and use a fork to mash them.
4. Place cashews in a food processor and pulse a few times. Add them to the large bowl.
5. Remove flax water from refrigerator and add to the large bowl. Mix well.
6. Form patties. You should have about 12.
7. Place on parchment paper.
8. Bake for 20 minutes. Then flip the patties and bake for an additional 15 minutes.
9. Allow cooling before removing patties.
10. Enjoy on a bun, over a salad, and with your favorite toppings.

Nutritional Information Per Serving: 280 Calories, 7 grams of Fat, 41 grams of Carbs, 13 grams of Protein

Time: 10 minutes

Serving Size: 3 servings

Ingredients:

- 1 15-oz can chickpeas, drained and rinsed
- 1 medium dill pickle, chopped
- 1 celery stalk, roughly chopped
- 2 tablespoons vegan mayo
- ½ tablespoon soy sauce

Directions:

1. In a bowl, use a fork to mash chickpeas. You can have a smooth texture or leave some beans whole.
2. Add in remaining ingredients and stir.
3. Place mixture in the refrigerator until ready to be consumed.

Note: This recipe should be served over a bed of lettuce, with crackers, or as a sandwich.

Dinner Ten - Instant Pot Pasta

Nutritional Information Per Serving: 325 Calories, 4 grams of Fat, 60 grams of Carbs, 18 grams of Protein

Time: 20 minutes

Serving Size: 5 servings

Ingredients:

- 1 tablespoon olive oil

- 1 small onion, diced
- 1 tablespoon garlic, minced
- 2 cups lentils, cooked
- 2 cups water
- 8 oz spaghetti
- 1 jar marinara sauce (25.5) ounces

Directions:

1. Press the sauté button on instant pot.
2. When hot add olive oil, onion, and garlic. Cook for 4 minutes. Stir occasionally.
3. Add salt, pepper, and cooked lentils. Stir.
4. Turn off the sauté.
5. Pour in water and use a spatula to make sure nothing is sticking to the bottom.
6. Break the noodles in half, and add to instant pot.
7. Pour marinara sauce over everything and close the cover. Don't stir.
8. Set instant pot to high pressure and cook for 9 minutes.
9. Do a quick release and then stir everything together. Enjoy!

Dinner Eleven - Peanut Tofu with Rice

Nutritional Information Per Serving: 460 Calories, 20 grams of Fat, 42 grams of Carbs, 19 grams of Protein

Time: 30 minutes

Serving Size: 3 servings

Ingredients:

Tofu:
- 1 block of tofu, extra-firm (vacuum sealed if possible)
- 1 tablespoon soy sauce
- 1 tablespoon cornstarch

Rice:

- ½ cup rice, dry
- ¼ cup canned coconut milk
- ¾ cup water
- sea salt to preference

Sauce:

- ¼ cup peanut butter
- ½ cup canned coconut milk
- 1 tablespoon soy sauce
- 1 teaspoon ginger, grater
- 1 teaspoon garlic, minced
- 1 tablespoon lime juice

Directions:

1. Press tofu and remove as much water as possible if the pack is not vacuum sealed.
2. Preheat oven to 400 Fahrenheit or 204 Celsius. Line a baking sheet with parchment paper and spray with oil.
3. Slice tofu into medium-sized cubes. Place them into a large bowl.
4. Add soy sauce and stir gently, followed by the cornstarch.
5. Place tofu cubes onto baking sheet and cook for 25 minutes. The tofu should appear crispy and golden brown.
6. In a pot, add rice, coconut milk, water, and salt. Bring water to a boil.
7. Turn to low heat and simmer the rice for 18 minutes.
8. In a large pan, add all the sauce ingredients and simmer over medium heat. Stir frequently. Allow the sauce to simmer for 10 minutes.
9. Add the tofu to the sauce and serve over rice!

Dinner Twelve - Spicy Tahini Pasta

Nutritional Information Per Serving: 325 Calories, 7 grams of Fat, 56 grams of Carbs, 15 grams of Protein

Time: 25 minutes

Serving Size: 4 servings

Ingredients:

For the Sauce:
- ¼ cup tahini
- ½ water
- ½ habanero pepper, seeded
- 1 tablespoon garlic, minced
- ½ lemon, juiced
- sea salt and pepper to preference

For the Pasta
- 8 ounces linguini pasta, cooked
- 2 cups green peas, steamed
- 4 cups mushrooms, sliced and sautéed
- a dab of oil for frying

Directions:

1. Prepare noodles and peas according to their packages and set aside.
2. In a pan, sauté mushrooms over medium heat for five minutes or until soft. Use a dab of oil if necessary.
3. In a separate pan, add garlic and habanero peppers. Sauté for 3 minutes.
4. Add all the sauce ingredients, including garlic and peppers, to a blender. Blend until smooth.
5. Add the sauce to the pan containing mushrooms. Stir.
6. Add in pasta and stir to combine all ingredients.
7. Enjoy and serve warm!

Dinner Thirteen - Sushi Bowl

Nutritional Information Per Serving: 600 Calories, 24 grams of Fat, 80 grams of Carbs, 17 grams of Protein

Time: 50 minutes

Serving Size: 4 servings

Ingredients:

For the Rice:
- 2 cups of rice, uncooked
- 1 sheet dried nori
- 3 tablespoons rice vinegar
- 2 teaspoons soy sauce
- 1 tablespoon sugar
- Himalayan salt to preference

For the Sauce:
- ⅓ cup vegan mayo
- 2 tablespoons sriracha

For the Toppings:

- 2 cups edamame, frozen
- 2 large carrots, shredded
- 1 avocado, pitted and sliced
- 1 cucumber, sliced
- pickled ginger (optional)

Directions:

1. Prepare rice using instructions on packaging.
2. In a small saucepan add rice vinegar, soy sauce, sugar, and salt. Simmer over medium heat until the sugar dissolves. Pour into rice and mix.
3. Warm the nori sheet in a large skillet over medium heat. This will allow the sheet to get crispy so you can crumble it into the sushi bowl. This should take about five to seven minutes.
4. Crumble the nori into the rice and stir.
5. Cook edamame by placing them into a pot of boiling water. Cook until they are tender and warmed through. Drain and set aside.
6. Add all the sauce ingredients into a bowl and whisk until well blended.
7. Assemble the bowls. Placing rice, toppings, and sauce into individual bowls.

Nutritional Information Per Serving: 315 Calories, 11 grams of Fat, 40 grams of Carbs, 9 grams of Protein

Time: 40 minutes

Serving Size: 6 servings

Ingredients:

- ½ tablespoon olive oil
- 1 medium onion, diced
- 1 tablespoon garlic, minced
- one small can mushrooms, sliced
- ½ tablespoon soy sauce
- 3.5 oz fresh spinach
- 1½ cups marinara sauce
- 6 lasagna noodles
- 1⅔ cups hummus
- 7 oz vegan cheese
- sea salt and pepper to preference

Directions:

1. Preheat oven to 360 Fahrenheit or 180 Celsius.
2. Cook lasagna noodles using directions on the packaging. Cook to al dente and drain when finished.
3. In a 9 x 6 baking dish, add ½ cup of marinara sauce to the bottom. Spread evenly.
4. In a pan, heat olive oil over medium heat. Add onion, garlic, and mushrooms.
5. After 4 minutes, add in soy sauce and spinach.
6. Turn off heat and add hummus/any additional spices. Stir.
7. Lay noodles on a flat surface and use ¼ hummus to spread onto each noodle.
8. Roll up each lasagna noodle and place it seam side down in the baking dish.
9. Pour remaining marinara over the top and sprinkle cheese. Bake for 25 minutes.

Nutritional Information Per Serving: 335 Calories, 12 grams of Fat, 47 grams of Carbs, 12 grams of Protein

Time: 30 minutes

Serving Size: 6 servings

Ingredients:

For the Sauce:
- 1 cup raw cashews, soaked
- ¾ cup water
- 1 tablespoon vinegar

For the Pasta:
- 10 oz penne pasta
- 1 small onion, chopped
- 16 oz mushrooms of choice
- 2 tablespoons garlic, minced
- 3 tablespoons flour
- 2 cups vegetable broth
- 2 teaspoons Dijon mustard
- sea salt and pepper to taste

Directions:

1. Cook pasta using instructions on packaging. Drain and set aside.
2. Soak cashews in boiling hot water for 5 minutes.
3. Add all the sauce ingredients into a high-powered blended and blend until creamy.
4. In a large pan, add mushrooms and onions. Cook over medium heat.
5. Stir in garlic, flour, vegetable broth, mustard, and spices.
6. Bring contents to a boil and then simmer for 5 minutes.
7. Add sauce and pasta. Stir.
8. Simmer for an additional 3 minutes, and serve warm.

Nutritional Information Per Serving: 255 Calories, 6 grams of Fat, 45 grams of Carbs, 7 grams of Protein

Time: 1 hour and 20 minutes

Serving Size: 3 servings

Ingredients:

- 1 large eggplant
- 1 tablespoon olive oil
- 1 medium onion, chopped
- ½ red bell pepper, seeded and chopped
- 1 teaspoon cumin seeds
- 1 teaspoon coriander
- ½ teaspoon turmeric
- 1 teaspoon garlic, minced
- 1 tablespoon ginger, grated
- 1 15-oz can tomatoes
- 1 15-oz can chickpeas
- 1 cup water
- ¼ cup parsley
- 4 cups rice, cooked
- sea salt and pepper to preference

Directions:

1. Preheat oven to 400 Fahrenheit or 205 Celsius.
2. Place eggplant on baking sheet and prick the outside for better cooking. Bake for 50 minutes.
3. Chop eggplant into medium to small pieces.
4. In a large skillet, add olive oil, onions, and peppers. Cook over medium heat.
5. Add in all spices.
6. Add tomatoes, chickpeas, eggplant, and water. Simmer on low heat for 20 minutes.
7. Stir in parsley and serve with rice!

Nutritional Information Per Serving: 213 Calories, 1 gram of Fat, 41 grams of Carbs, 10 grams of Protein

Time: 40 minutes

Serving Size: 2 pizza crusts, 2 servings

Ingredients:

- 1 cup hot water
- 1 envelope instant yeast
- 1 tablespoon sugar
- 2¾ cup whole wheat flour
- ¼ cup nutritional yeast
- 1 teaspoon salt

Directions:

1. Preheat oven to 425 Fahrenheit or 218 Celsius. Lightly grease two large baking pans.
2. In a large bowl, combine hot water, yeast, and sugar. Whisk the dough together and set aside for 5 minutes.
3. Add flour, nutritional yeast, and salt. Knead dough on a non-stick surface until the mixture is smooth.
4. Cut the dough into even halves.
5. Roll out the dough using fingers or baking pin.
6. Place the dough onto the baking pans.
7. Add desired toppings and sauce.
8. Bake for 8 to 10 minutes or until the crust is to your liking.

Nutritional Information Per Serving: 365 Calories, 15 grams of Fat, 47 grams of Carbs, 8 grams of Protein

Time: 30 minutes

Serving Size: 6 servings

Ingredients:

- 2 tablespoons avocado oil
- 1 medium onion, sliced
- 1 tablespoon garlic, minced
- 3 carrots, peeled and shredded
- 3 pounds potatoes, peeled and in chunks
- 3 cups vegetable broth
- 1 15-oz can coconut milk
- sea salt and pepper to preference

Directions:

1. In a large soup pot, add all ingredients including coconut milk.
2. Bring contents to a boil and then reduce to low heat. Simmer for 25 minutes.
3. Place contents carefully into a blender and blend until smooth.
4. Return contents back to pot and add coconut milk.
5. Simmer for additional 2 minutes an enjoy warm.

Dinner Nineteen - Mac n' Cheese

Nutritional Information Per Serving: 305 Calories, 11 grams of Fat, 40 grams of Carbs, 12 grams of Protein

Time: 20 minutes

Serving Size: 4 servings

Ingredients:

- ¾ cup raw cashews
- ½ cup vegetable broth
- ½ lemon, juiced
- ¼ cup nutritional yeast

- ¼ teaspoon turmeric
- ¼ teaspoon onion powder
- 6 ounces pasta of choice
- sea salt and pepper to preference

Directions:

1. Pour boiling hot water over cashews and soak for at least 5 minutes.
2. Cook pasta using instructions on packaging.
3. In a blender, process cashews, vegetable broth, water, lemon juice, nutritional yeast, and spices. Blend until smooth.
4. When pasta is done, drain and return to pot along with cashew sauce.
5. Allow everything to simmer for an additional 5 minutes stirring frequently.

Dinner Twenty - Sesame Chickpeas

Nutritional Information Per Serving: 300 Calories, 7 grams of Fat, 42 grams of Carbs, 10 grams of Protein

Time: 15 minutes

Serving Size: 3 servings

Ingredients:

- 1 15-oz can chickpeas, drained and rinsed
- 2 teaspoons of garlic, minced
- ½ tablespoon coconut oil
- 1 tablespoon sesame oil
- 3 tablespoons soy sauce
- 1 tablespoon maple syrup
- 1 teaspoon rice vinegar
- 1 tablespoon vegetable broth
- sea salt and pepper to preference

Directions:

1. In a saucepan, add coconut oil and garlic. Simmer over medium heat for 2 minutes.

2. Add soy sauce, sesame oil, maple syrup, rice vinegar, and vegetable oil. Mix well.
3. Cook on low heat for 4 minutes or until bubbles form.
4. Add in chickpeas and stir.
5. Cook on low heat until sticky texture is achieved.

Note: This recipe is best served over broccoli, quinoa, or rice.

Dinner Twenty-One - Buffalo Bites

Nutritional Information Per Serving: 245 Calories, 22 grams of Fat, 32 grams of Carbs, 7 grams of Protein

Time: 1 hour

Serving Size: 4 servings

Ingredients:

For the Sauce:
- ½ cup vegan mayo
- 1 teaspoon dill
- 1 teaspoon parsley

For the Bites:
- 1 head of cauliflower, in florets
- ¾ cup chickpea flour
- ¾ cup almond milk, unsweetened
- ¼ cup water
- 2 teaspoons of garlic powder
- 2 teaspoons smoked paprika
- 1 cup panko bread crumbs
- 1 cup hot sauce
- 1 tablespoon olive oil

Directions:

1. Preheat oven to 350 Fahrenheit or 177 Celsius. Line a baking sheet with parchment paper.
2. In a large bowl, combine flour, milk, water, garlic powder, smoked paprika, salt, and pepper. Toss to coat everything evenly.
3. Dip florets into batter and coat the entire floret evenly.
4. Place breadcrumbs into a bowl.
5. Roll each floret into the breadcrumbs and place onto lined baking sheet.
6. Bake for 25 minutes.
7. Combine hot sauce and olive oil and pour over florets. Stir florets to evenly coat.
8. Bake for an additional 20 minutes and remove from oven to cool off a bit.
9. Combine all sauce ingredients in a bowl and serve with bites!

Dinner Twenty-Two - Black Bean Soup

Nutritional Information Per Serving: 305 Calories, 7 grams of Fat, 43 grams of Carbs, 10 grams of Protein

Time: 20 minutes

Serving Size: 8 servings

Ingredients:

- 3 tablespoons avocado oil
- 1 large onion, roughly chopped
- 2 tablespoons garlic, minced
- 1 teaspoon ground cumin
- 2 15-oz cans black beans, drained and rinsed
- 1½ cups corn
- 1 28-oz can diced tomatoes
- 1 quart vegetable stock
- 2 teaspoons cayenne pepper (optional)
- sea salt and pepper to preference

Directions:

1. In a large soup pot, add olive oil, onion, and garlic. Cook over medium heat for 4 minutes.
2. Add beans, corn, tomatoes, and vegetable stock. Boil and then reduce heat to medium low.
3. Add seasonings.
4. Simmer on low for 15 minutes and serve with your favorite toppings.

Dinner Twenty-Three - Lentil Bolognese

Nutritional Information Per Serving: 250 Calories, 6 grams of Fat, grams of Carbs, 10 grams of Protein

Time: 55 minutes

Serving Size: 6 servings

Ingredients:
- 1 large onion
- 2 tablespoons garlic, minced
- 2 carrots
- 2 celery stalks
- 1 portobello mushroom
- 1 red bell pepper
- 2 tablespoons avocado oil
- ¾ cup red wine
- 2 cups lentils, cooked
- 2 cups crushed tomatoes
- 2 bay leaves
- 1 tablespoon Italian seasoning
- 1 tablespoon lemon juice
- ¾ cup water
- salt & pepper to taste
- handful of parsley, finely chopped

Directions:

1. Add onion, garlic, carrots, celery, mushrooms, salt, and pepper to a food processor and pulse into small pieces.
2. In a large pan, sauté the vegetables over medium-high heat. Use oil as needed to prevent burning. Sauté for 15 minutes and stir frequently.
3. Add in wine and cook over medium heat until the wine evaporates.
4. Add lentils, crushed tomatoes, and all seasonings. Mix well.
5. Lower heat to low, and add water. Simmer for additional 20 minutes.
6. Remove bay leaves.
7. Pulse the sauce with a blender or serve as is. Add in parsley when serving.

Note: This recipe is best served over pasta or rice.

Dinner Twenty-Four - Instant Pot Wild Rice Soup

Nutritional Information Per Serving: 375 Calories, 15 grams of Fat, 45 grams of Carbs, 12 grams of Protein

Time: 55 minutes (overnight recipe)

Serving Size: 4 servings

Ingredients:

- ½ cup raw cashews, soaked overnight
- 1 cup water
- 1 teaspoon nutritional yeast
- 2 tablespoons olive oil
- 1 large onion, chopped
- 1 tablespoon garlic, minced
- 1 carrot, chopped
- 1 celery stalk, chopped
- 1 cup mushrooms, sliced
- 1 cup wild rice
- 2 teaspoons rosemary
- 1 bay leaf

- 5 cups vegetable broth
- sea salt and black pepper to preference

Directions:

1. In a high-speed blender add cashews, water, and nutritional yeast. Blend for one minute or until creamy.
2. Set Instant Pot to sauté and add olive oil, garlic, carrot, celery, and mushrooms. Cook for 5 minutes.
3. Add rice, rosemary, bay leaf, salt, and pepper. Mix well.
4. Add broth.
5. Seal instant pot and set to pressure cook on manual for 35 minutes.
6. Allow the pressure to release naturally for 10 minutes. Turn the lid to venting to finish releasing pressure.
7. Stir cashew mixture into soup and serve warm!

Dinner Twenty-Five - Fried Rice

Nutritional Information Per Serving: 450 Calories, 7 grams of Fat, 65 grams of Carbs, 17 grams of Protein

Time: 30 minutes

Serving Size: 4 servings

Ingredients:
For the Tofu:
- 2 teaspoons of coconut oil
- ½ pack tofu, medium firm
- ¼ teaspoon turmeric powder
- ¼ teaspoon soy sauce

For the Rice:
- 1 cup brown rice
- 2 teaspoons of coconut oil
- 1 onion
- 1 teaspoon garlic, minced

- 1 large carrot, diced
- 1 celery stalk, diced
- ½ cup peas, cooked
- 1 tablespoon soy sauce
- 1 teaspoon sesame oil
- 1 teaspoon sriracha

Directions:
1. Heat two teaspoons of coconut oil in a medium pan, over medium heat.
2. Crumble in tofu. Cook for five to six minutes.
3. Add turmeric and soy sauce. Mix well.
4. Heat remaining two teaspoons of oil in the pan and add the onion. Cook for three minutes.
5. Add garlic, carrots, and celery. Cook for five minutes.
6. Add peas, rice, soy sauce, sesame oil, sriracha, and tofu. Mix until everything is combined evenly.
7. Let the mixture simmer over low heat for three minutes.
8. Remove from heat and serve warm or cold.

Dinner Twenty-Six - Seitan

Nutritional information per serving:

Calories	107g	Carbs	5g	Iron	8%
Sugar	0g	Protein	21g	Calcium	4%
Fiber	1g	Fat	5g		

What You Need:

Dough:
- Vital wheat gluten - 1 cup (200g)
- Whole wheat or chickpea flour—0.25 cup (50g)
- Water - 1 cup (236ml)

Broth:

- Low sodium vegetable broth - 6 cups (1,416ml)
- Soy sauce - 0.25 cup (60ml)
- Optional flavorings of your choice (below)

Chicken flavor:	Pork flavor:	Beef flavor:
Nutritional yeast flakes (.25 cup)	2 tbsp maple syrup (2 tbsp)	Dry red wine (1.5 cup)
White wine vinegar (1.5 tsp)	Apple cider vinegar (2 tbsp)	Vegan Worcestershire sauce (2 tbsp)
Poultry seasoning (1.5 tsp)	Liquid smoke (2 tsp)	Dried thyme (1 tsp)
Onion powder (1 tsp)	Smoked paprika (2 tsp)	Onion powder (1.5 tsp)
Garlic powder (1.5 tsp)	Onion powder (1tsp)	Garlic powder (1.5 tsp)
Liquid smoke (1.5 tsp)	Garlic powder (1tsp)	Black pepper (1.5 tsp)

What to Do:

1. In a mixing bowl of medium size, stir together the wheat gluten and flour. Add some dried seasoning here if you like—salt, pepper, garlic powder, etc.
2. Slowly add the water to the dry elements and stir until a soft dough begins to form. With your hands, use the ball of dough to pick up loose dried ingredients on the edge of the bowl and knead the dough until all parts are mixed.
3. Transfer the dough onto a work surface and knead with your hands for five to ten minutes. The dough will become stringy and firm. If the dough is too moist, sprinkle more gluten and knead it into the mixture. Once you've thoroughly kneaded the dough, allow it to rest for five minutes.
4. To create the broth, add all the ingredients to a large pot and bring it to a boil. The dough will double in size, so ensure the pot you use has ample room. Once boiling, lower the heat and allow the broth to come to a low simmer.
5. Cut the dough into four large pieces. You can also cut into small strips or chunks. The pieces will stick together slightly as the dough simmers.

6. Add the dough to the simmering broth. Allow to simmer, uncovered, for one hour. Watch closely and do not allow the broth to boil. It is essential to keep the broth at a low simmer for the whole hour.
7. Remove from the heat by placing it in a strainer to cool for five to ten minutes.
8. Once cooled, you can handle the seitan. Cut it into smaller pieces and use immediately or keep in the fridge for up to five days. You can also leave seitan in the freezer for up to one month.
9. You can enjoy the seitan as-is or cook it further by frying in a pan with more seasoning, baking with another recipe, or adding to a soup.

Dinner Twenty-Seven - Buddha Bowl With Peanut Tofu

Nutritional information per serving:

Calories	496	Carbs	58g	Sodium	33%
Sugar	22g	Protein	19g	Cholesterol	0%
Fiber	7g	Fat	24g		

What You Need:
- 14 oz extra firm tofu - 14 oz (396g), pressed
- Sweet potato - 1, large, cubed
- Brown basmati rice, or any whole grain - 0.75 cup (150g)

Peanut Sauce:
- Fresh ginger - 3 slices, peeled, roughly the size of a quarter
- Garlic clove - 1, large, sliced thin
- Peanut butter - 0.25 cup (50ml)
- Orange juice - 0.5 orange, squeezed
- Soy sauce or coconut aminos - 2 tbsp (30ml)
- Maple syrup - 3 tsp (15ml)
- Dash of hot sauce (Sriracha is perfect)

- Pinch of sea salt

Veggies:
- Shredded carrots - 2 cups (400g)
- Shredded cabbage - 2 cups (400g)
- Shredded beets - 2 cups (400g)
- Snap peas - 1cup (200g)
- Radishes - 0.5 cup (100g), thinly sliced
- Avocados - 2, large
- Microgreens (bean sprouts of alfalfa) - 1 cup (200g)

What to Do:

1. Ensure that your oven is Preheated to 425 degrees Fahrenheit
2. While the oven is warming, press the tofu and cut into two-inch cubes or slices. The cubed tofu will be placed in a single layer on one half of a baking sheet lined with parchment paper and sprinkle with salt.
3. Wash the sweet potato and cut into .75 inch cubes. Place the sweet potato on the other side of the baking sheet. Drizzle the sweet potato with olive oil and sprinkle lightly with salt and toss to coat. Spread evenly over half of the baking sheet.
4. Prepare the peanut sauce by placing all peanut sauce ingredients in a blender and blend until smooth. Save half of the sauce for the dressing. Use half the sauce to coat the tofu. Pour over tofu and brush the tops and sides of each piece.
5. Place in the hot oven and cook for twenty-five to thirty minutes.
6. Cook the rice or whole-grain according to package orders—or if you have prepared some earlier skip this step and simply warm in the oven for ten minutes as the tofu cooks.
7. Prep the veggies. Use a mandolin to shred the vegetables quickly or chop each on into bite-sized pieces.
8. Once the tofu has cooked and the sweet potatoes are tender, you can assemble the bowls. Layer grains, veggies, tofu and sweet potato into four individual bowls. Drizzle with the rest of the saved peanut sauce and top with microgreens and diced avocado.

This recipe will give you six servings.

Nutritional information per serving:

Calories	31g	Carbs	7g	Sodium	35%
Sugar	3g	Protein	10g	Vitamin A	80%
Fiber	2g	Fat	4g		

What You Need:

Broth:

- Low sodium vegetable broth - 8 cups (1,888ml)
- Water - 3 cups (708ml)
- Garlic - 4 cloves, chopped
- Onion - 1, medium, chopped
- Soy sauce or coconut aminos - 2 tbsp (30ml)
- Ground clove - 1 tbsp (15g)
- Fresh ginger - 1 inch, peeled and cut into quarter-sized slices
- Cinnamon - 1 stick, optional
- Whole star anise - 3, optional

Soup:

- Rice noodles (1 package)
- Sautéed or baked tofu - 14 oz (396g)
- Basil, Cilantro and Mint—fresh
- Green onions—fresh
- Hot peppers—sliced
- Mung bean sprouts
- Mushrooms—sautéed
- Carrots—shredded
- Cabbage—shredded
- Peanuts—toasted
- Hot sauce
- Lime wedges

What to Do:

1. In a medium pot, add the broth, water, garlic, onion, ginger, and spices. Bring to a low simmer, then cover and let simmer for twenty to thirty minutes. Taste and add soy sauce or aminos as needed.
2. While the broth simmers, cook the rice noodles according to the orders on the package.
3. Prepare tofu by pressing and either sautéing or baking (see "How to maketofu taste great)
4. Prepare the vegetables and arrange in individual serving dishes.
5. Once everything is ready, provide six serving bowls and allow guests to build their own meals by layering noodles, broth, and their choice of vegetables and garnishes.

Dinner Twenty-Nine - Vegan Pizza

This recipe will give you four servings.

Nutritional information per serving:

Calories	395	Carbs	59g	Sodium	20%
Sugar	19g	Protein	15g	Vitamin C	25%
Fiber	8g	Fat	16g		

What You Need:

Sauce:

- Tomato sauce - 30 oz can (850g)
- Basil - 1.5 tsp (7.5g)
- Oregano - 1.5 tsp (7.5g)
- Garlic powder - 1.5 tsp (7.5g)
- Sugar - 1 tsp (5g)

Toppings:

- Red pepper - 1 cup (200g), sliced
- Orange pepper= 1 cup (200g), sliced
- Green pepper - 1 cup (200g), sliced
- Red onion - 0.5 cup (100g), sliced
- White mushrooms - 2 cups (400g), sliced
- Basil - 1.5 tsp (7.5g)
- Oregano - 1.5 tsp (7.5g)
- Garlic powder - 1.5 tsp (7.5g)

Non-dairy shredded cheese - 1 cup (200g) Daiya makes a good option for pizza.
Frozen, premade vegan pizza crust. Trader Joe's makes a great option.

What to Do:

1. Ensure your oven is Preheated to 425 degrees Fahrenheit (218 Celsius)
2. In a large skillet heat some olive oil on medium heat, once hot add all the peppers and onion. Season with salt and herbs, stir, and cook for ten to fifteen minutes until soft and lightly charred. Add the mushrooms and cook for two to three minutes then set aside.
3. Prepare the sauce by mixing the tomato sauce, herbs, and sugar in a bowl. Season lightly with salt and adjust the seasonings to your preference.
4. Lay some parchment paper on a flat surface, like a large cutting board. The dough will go in the oven on the parchment paper so you can use any flat surface to transfer to the oven as it won't be going in with the pizza. Place the dough on the parchment paper and begin to assemble the pizza.
5. Spread a layer of tomato sauce on the dough. Spread the sautéed veggies on top of the sauce and sprinkle with non-dairy cheese.
6. Use the flat surface to transfer the pizza with the parchment paper onto the oven rack directly. The parchment paper will prevent anything from falling through, and the direct heat will create a perfectly crisp pizza crust.
7. Bake for seventeen to twenty minutes, until the edges look crisp and golden brown.

This recipe will give you four servings.

Nutritional information per serving:

Calories	520	Carbs	74g	Sodium	10%
Sugar	7g	Protein	22g	Magnesium	15%
Fiber	6g	Fat	15g		

What You Need:

- Eggless fettuccine noodles - 12 oz (340g)
- Unsweetened non-dairy milk - 2 cups (472ml)
- Non-dairy cream cheese - 4 oz (113g)
- Garlic - 6 cloves, minced
- Nutritional yeast - 3.5 tbsp (52g)
- Lemon zest - 1 tsp (5g), grated
- Olive oil - 2 tbsp (30ml)
- Fresh basil leaves - 0.25 cup (50g), chopped finely
- Salt and pepper to taste

What to Do:

1. Cook the noodles in a medium pot according to the orders on the package. Strain, reserving 1 cup of the pasta water. Set the noodles aside once cooked.
2. In a blender, add the non-dairy milk, cream cheese, nutritional yeast, lemon zest, salt & pepper. Blend until creamy and smooth.
3. In a large skillet, cook the garlic over medium heat for one minute. Add the cheese mixture from the blender and ½ cup of the reserved pasta water. Bring the sauce to a low simmer and cook until it becomes thick and creamy. Approximately seven to eight minutes.
4. Remove from the heat and add the cooked noodles to the skillet with the sauce, stir to combine. If you find the sauce is too thick, you can slowly stir in the rest

of the reserved pasta water 1 tbsp at a time. If you are adding additional vegetables of a plant-based protein, stir them in now.

5. Serve in individual dishes and top with nutritional yeast or chopped fresh herbs.

Dinner Thirty-One - Southwest Stuffed Peppers

This recipe will give you four servings.

Nutritional information per serving:

Calories	520	Carbs	74g	Sodium	10%
Sugar	7g	Protein	22g	Magnesium	15%
Fiber	6g	Fat	15g		

What You Need:

- Olive oil - 1 tbsp (15ml)
- Garlic - 4 cloves, minced
- Onion - 1, small, minced
- Bell peppers - 3, large, cut in half, seeds removed
- Tomato - 2, large, chopped
- Black beans - 1 15 oz (425g) can, drained and rinsed
- Corn kernels - 1 6 oz (150g) can, drained and rinsed
- Chili powder - 1 tsp (5g)
- Salt and pepper to taste

Add Ons:
- Guacamole - 0.25 cup (50ml), optional
- Salsa =0.25 cup (50ml), optional
- Non-dairy cheese shreds—optional

What to Do:

1. Ensure your oven is preheated to 350 degrees Fahrenheit (180 degrees Celsius)

2. Place the halved bell peppers in a square roasting pan, drizzle with olive oil and rub on to cover the outer surface of peppers. Cook in the oven for fifteen to twenty minutes. They should be slightly browned and soft but still holding their shape. When done cooking, remove from oven and allow to cool.

3. While the peppers are cooking, add the onion and garlic to a pan and sauté on medium heat for one minute. Add the black beans and chili powder to the pan, use a small splash of water, roughly a tablespoon to keep the beans from sticking. Mash the beans gently with a fork, leaving some whole still.

4. Stir in the corn and diced tomato. Season with salt and pepper and taste. Adjust by adding more chili powder if needed.

5. Scoop the bean mixture evenly into the cooked pepper halves. Place back in the oven and cook for five to 8 minutes.

6. Serve as-is or with a creamy cashew sauce, guacamole, salsa. You can also sprinkle non-dairy cheese on the mixture before placing it in the oven for the final five to eight minutes of cooking.

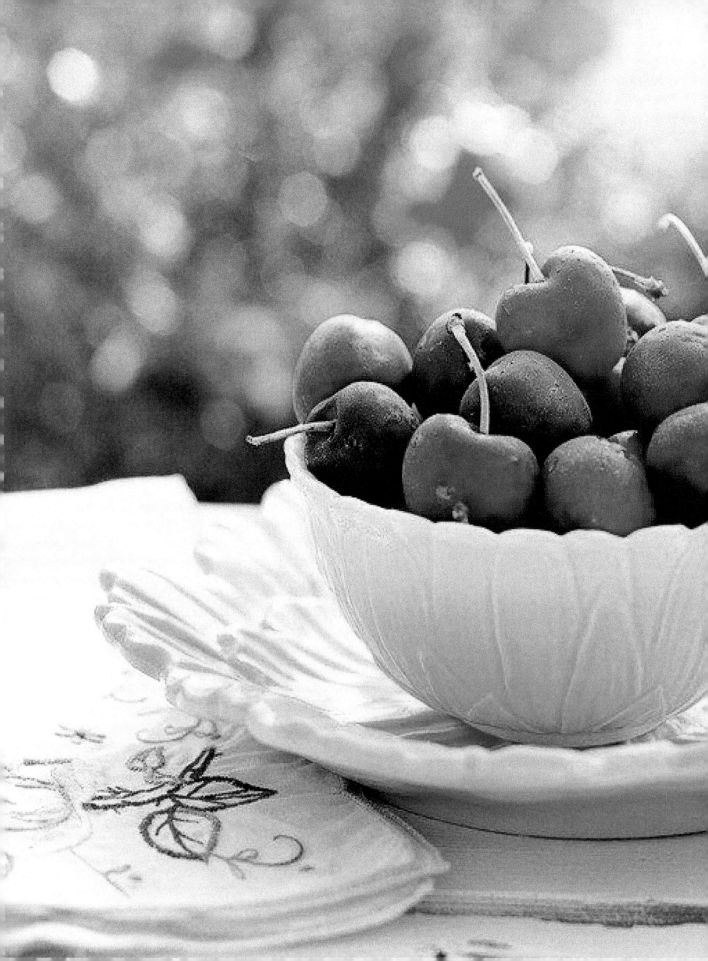

Chapter 10: Snacks & Dessert Recipes

Snack 1 - Spinach and Artichoke Dip

Nutritional Information Per Serving: 75 Calories, 6 grams of Fat, 5 grams of Carbs, 3 grams of Protein

Time: 20 minutes

Serving Size: 10 servings

Ingredients:

- 1 tablespoon avocado oil
- 3 cloves garlic, diced
- 12 oz marinated artichoke hearts
- 4 cups baby spinach, chopped
- ¼ cup vegan mayo
- 8 oz vegan cream cheese
- ½ teaspoon onion powder
- sea salt and black pepper to preference

Directions:

1. Preheat oven to 400 Fahrenheit or 205 Celsius.
2. Heat the avocado oil in a pan over medium heat. Add garlic, artichoke hearts, and spinach. Simmer for three minutes.
3. Add cream cheese, mayo, onion powder, salt, and pepper. Mix well.
4. Add the mixture to a baking dish and place under the broiler for five minutes.
5. Remove and enjoy warm.

Note: This recipe is best served with crackers or tortilla chips. This recipe is excellent to bring to parties.

Nutritional Information Per Serving: 190 Calories, 16 grams of Fat, 10 grams of Carbs, 6 grams of Protein

Time: 40 minutes

Serving Size: 10 servings

Ingredients:

- 2 cups raw cashews
- 1 cup water
- 3 tablespoons lemon juice
- 2 teaspoons onion powder
- 1 teaspoon garlic powder
- 1 cup buffalo/hot sauce
- 14 oz artichoke hearts, drained
- sea salt and black pepper to preference

Directions:

1. Preheat oven to 375 Fahrenheit or 190 degrees Celsius.
2. Pour boiling hot water over cashews and allow them to soak for 5 minutes. Drain and place in blender when finished.
3. Add water, lemon juice, garlic powder, onion powder, salt and pepper to the blender containing the cashews. Blend until smooth.
4. Add buffalo sauce and artichoke hearts to the blender. Pulse until the artichoke hearts are broken down. You'll want to leave some texture to the dip.
5. Transfer to baking dish and bake for 30 minutes.

Note: This recipe is best served with celery sticks, carrot sticks, tortilla chips, crackers, or bread.

Nutritional Information Per Serving: 250 Calories, 6 grams of Fat, grams of Carbs, 10 grams of Protein

Time: 45 minutes

Serving Size: 6 servings

Ingredients:

- 4 medium potatoes
- 2 tablespoons avocado oil
- 2 teaspoons of garlic powder
- 2 teaspoons onion powder
- 1 teaspoon smoked paprika
- Himalayan salt and pepper to preference

Directions:

1. Preheat oven to 425 Fahrenheit or 218 Celsius. Grease a large baking pan with a dab of oil.
2. Clean potatoes and remove dirt.
3. Slice potatoes in half and then into wedges.
4. In a large Ziplock bag, place potatoes and all other ingredients. Shake the bag to evenly coat the potatoes.
5. Spread potatoes oven baking pan and bake for 35 minutes. Flip and stir the wedges halfway through.
6. Remove wedges when golden brown and tender. Serve warm with your favorite vegan sauce.

Snack Four - Dill Hummus

Nutritional Information Per Serving: 105 Calories, 6 grams of Fat, 12 grams of Carbs, 5 grams of Protein

Time: 5 minutes

Serving Size: 6 servings

Ingredients:

- 1 15-oz can chickpeas, rinsed and drained
- ¼ cup lemon juice
- ¼ cup fresh dill, chopped
- 3 tablespoons tahini
- 2 tablespoons water
- sea salt and black pepper to taste

Directions:

1. Add all ingredients to a blender and blend until smooth. Omit the water for a thicker consistency.

Note: This recipe is best served with veggie sticks, crackers, pita chips, or tortilla chips. This can also be a great addition to salads, sandwiches, and other dishes.

Snack Five - Latte Pudding

Nutritional Information Per Serving: 200 Calories, 14 grams of Fat, 15 grams of Carbs, 5 grams of Protein

Time: 15 minutes (overnight recipe)

Serving Size: 4 servings

Ingredients:
- 1¼ cups water
- 2 chai tea bags
- ⅓ cup raw cashews, soaked overnight
- ½ teaspoon vanilla extract
- 2 tablespoons maple syrup
- ½ teaspoon cinnamon
- ¼ teaspoon nutmeg
- ¼ cup chia seeds
- pinch of salt

Directions:

1. Steep the chai tea bags in water for five minutes. Throw away tea bags when finished.
2. Add chai tea, cashews, vanilla, maple syrup, cinnamon, salt, and nutmeg to a high-speed blender. Blend until smooth.
3. Pour mixture to a bowl containing the chia seeds and whisk to mix everything well. Leave the mixture in the refrigerator overnight to firm up.
4. Serve with favorite toppings or fruit.

Snack Six - Peanut Butter

Nutritional Information Per Serving: 178 Calories, 15 grams of Fat, 5 grams of Carbs, 8 grams of Protein

Time: 5 minutes

Serving Size: 14 servings

Ingredients:

- 3 cups raw or roasted peanuts
- 1 teaspoon vanilla
- sea salt to preference

Directions:

1. Add all ingredients to a high-speed food processor and blend until smooth. This may take several minutes, and you may need to scrape the sides of the blender frequently.

Nutritional Information Per Serving (2 Scoops): 50 Calories, 2 grams of Fat, 4 grams of Carbs, 2 grams of Protein

Time: 25 minutes

Serving Size: 30 servings

Ingredients:
- 1 cup quinoa flour
- ½ cup sorghum flour
- ½ cup nutritional yeast
- ½ teaspoon Himalayan salt
- ½ cup kale, finely chopped
- 2 tablespoon olive oil
- ⅔ cup cold water

Directions:

1. Preheat the oven to 450 Fahrenheit or 232 Celsius. Line a baking sheet with parchment paper.
2. Toast quinoa on the stove and stir frequently.
3. Allow the flour to cool for 5 minutes before adding to a food processor.
4. Add sorghum flour, nutritional yeast, and salt. Pulse a few times.
5. Add kale and pulse.
6. Add in oil and water until the dough starts to come together.
7. Remove the dough and form it into a ball. Let the dough rest for a few minutes.
8. Separate the dough into four pieces. Knead each piece with your hands.
9. Roll each part as thin as possible.
10. Transfer the dough onto the baking sheets after rolling.
11. Bake the crackers for 5 minutes on each side.
12. Turn the oven off but allow the crackers to stay in the oven for one or two hours to get crispy.
13. Remove from oven and allow cooking before breaking them into pieces.

Nutritional Information Per Serving: 300 Calories, 13 grams of Fat, 42 grams of Carbs, 8 grams of Protein

Time: 40 minutes

Serving Size: 9 servings

Ingredients:

- 1 15-oz can chickpeas, rinsed and drained
- ¾ cup brown sugar
- ⅓ cup creamy peanut butter
- 1 teaspoon vanilla extract
- ¼ cup almond flour
- ¼ teaspoon baking soda
- ½ teaspoon baking powder
- ¾ cup vegan chocolate chips
- pinch of Himalayan salt

Directions:

1. Preheat oven to 350 Fahrenheit or 177 Celsius. Line an 8 x 8 pan with parchment paper.
2. Add all ingredients to a food processor except for the chocolate chips. Blend until smooth.
3. Fold in half of the chocolate chips.
4. Pour batter into the pan. Sprinkle the rest of the chocolate chips on top.
5. Bake for 27 minutes.
6. Let the blondies cool before serving.

Nutritional Information Per Serving: 215 Calories, 16 grams of Fat, 22 grams of Carbs, 5 grams of Protein

Time: 30 minutes

Serving Size: 12 servings

Ingredients:

- 2 cups vegan chocolate chips
- ½ cup peanut butter
- 4 tablespoons powdered sugar
- pinch of salt

Directions:

1. Line muffin tray with paper liners. You will need 12 liners.
2. Microwave 1 cup of chocolate chips in a microwave-safe bowl for one minute.
3. Stir and repeat in five second increments to prevent burning. Stir frequently.
4. Scoop ½ tablespoon of the chocolate and place into each liner. Use a spoon to create an even surface and bring the chocolate up onto the sides of the liner.
5. Repeat step 4 until each liner is filled.
6. Freeze the muffin pan for 10 minutes.
7. In a bowl, add peanut butter, salt, and powdered sugar. Mix well until a dough is formed.
8. Remove pan from freezer and place a tablespoon of peanut butter into each cup. Press down on the dough with a spoon to create a smooth surface.
9. Freeze pan for additional 10 minutes.
10. Melt remaining chocolate chips. Spoon chocolate evenly over the now frozen peanut butter mixture.
11. Remove the liners and store in the refrigerator to prevent melting until ready to be consumed.

Nutritional Information Per Serving: 320 Calories, 16 grams of Fat, 42 grams of Carbs, 5 grams of Protein

Time: 1 minute

Serving Size: 1 serving

Ingredients:
- 2 tablespoons all-purpose flour
- 2 tablespoons cocoa powder
- 2 tablespoons sugar
- ¼ teaspoon baking powder
- 1 tablespoon coconut oil
- 3 tablespoons coconut milk
- ½ teaspoon pure vanilla extract
- 2 tablespoons vegan chocolate chips
- pinch of Himalayan salt

Directions:

1. In a microwave safe mug, add flour, cocoa powder, sugar, salt, and baking powder. Stir well.
2. Pour in the oil, milk, and vanilla into the mug. Mix well then add chocolate chips on top.
3. Microwave for 40 seconds and serve immediately.

Dessert Four - Ice Cream

Nutritional Information Per Serving (2 Scoops): 140 Calories, 15 grams of Fat, 4 grams of Carbs, 3 grams of Protein

Time: 5 minutes

Serving Size: 10 servings

Ingredients:

- 2 14-oz cans full-fat coconut milk
- ½ cup soaked cashews, raw
- ⅓ cup cocoa powder
- 1 teaspoon vanilla extract
- pinch of sea salt
- sweetener of choice

Directions:

1. In a blender, place all ingredients and blend until smooth.
2. Place the mixture in a plastic Ziploc bag and freeze until solid.
3. When ready to consume, allow the ice cream to thaw slightly before serving.

Dessert Five - Chocolate Chip Cookies

Nutritional Information Per Cookies: 130 Calories, 7 grams of Fat, 16 grams of Carbs, 1 grams of Protein

Time: 25 minutes

Serving Size: 36 cookies

Ingredients:

- ¾ cup coconut oil, melted
- ¾ cup sugar
- ¾ cup brown sugar
- ½ cup applesauce, unsweetened
- 2 teaspoons vanilla
- 2½ cups flour, all-purpose
- 1 teaspoon baking soda
- 1 teaspoon sea salt
- ½ teaspoon baking powder
- 1¼ cup vegan chocolate chips

Directions:

1. Preheat oven to 350 Fahrenheit or 177 Celsius. Line a baking sheet with parchment paper.
2. In a large bowl, add coconut oil, sugar, brown sugar, applesauce, and vanilla. Mix well.
3. Add in flour, baking soda, baking powder, and salt to form a dough.
4. Fold in chocolate chips.
5. Form the cookies. One tablespoon of dough should yield one cookie. Place the cookies two inches apart. Do not press them down. Leave them in a small ball.
6. Bake for 12 minutes or until edges are brown.
7. Allow the cookies to cool, and they will harden up a bit.
8. Serve with your favorite plant-based milk!

Dessert Six - Vanilla Cupcakes

Nutritional Information Per Serving (2 Scoops): 195 Calories, 10 grams of Fat, 25 grams of Carbs, 2 grams of Protein

Time: 20 minutes

Serving Size: 12 servings

Ingredients:
For the Cupcakes:
- 1 cup almond milk
- 1 tablespoon apple cider vinegar
- ¾ cup sugar
- ½ cup coconut oil
- 1 teaspoon vanilla extract
- 1½ cups flour, all-purpose
- 2 teaspoons baking powder
- pinch of salt

For the Frosting:
- ½ cup vegan butter, softened

- ¼ teaspoon vanilla extract
- 1½ cups powdered sugar
- 1 teaspoon almond milk

Directions:

1. Preheat oven to 350 Fahrenheit or 175 Celsius. Line a muffin tray with liners.
2. In a large bowl, add almond milk and vinegar. Stir and set aside for five minutes.
3. Using an electric mixer, beat the sugar, coconut oil, and vanilla into the bowl containing the almond milk/vinegar mixture.
4. Slowly add in flour, baking powder, and salt. Mix well but do not overmix.
5. Pour batter evenly throughout the liners.
6. Bake for 15 minutes.
7. Beat the frosting ingredients until fluffy.
8. Let the cupcakes cool for five minutes before transferring them to a wire rack.
9. Let the cupcakes cool completely before adding the frosting using your method of choice.

Dessert Seven - Edible Cookie Dough

Nutritional Information Per Serving: 80 Calories, 3 grams of Fat, 4 grams of Carbs, 3 grams of Protein

Time: 10 minutes

Serving Size: 1-2 servings

Ingredients:
- 1 cup almond flour, finely ground
- 3 tablespoons coconut butter, melted
- 3 tablespoons maple syrup
- 1 teaspoon vanilla extract
- ½ teaspoon ground cinnamon

- ¼ cup vegan chocolate chips
- pinch of sea salt

Directions:

1. Add all ingredients to a bowl and stir. Mix well and taste as you go. Adjust any flavors to your liking.
2. Store in the refrigerator.

Note: This recipe is great alone or with other desserts such as ice cream crumbled over cakes, or on top of smoothies.

Dessert Eight - Fat Bomb

Nutritional Information Per Serving (2 Scoops): 85 Calories, 9 grams of Fat, 25 grams of Carbs, 2 grams of Protein

Time: 5 minutes

Serving Size: 13 servings

Ingredients:
- ½ cup almond butter
- 2½ tablespoons coconut oil

Directions:

1. Combine both ingredients in a bowl and warm in the microwave until both ingredients are soft.
2. Pour into cupcake liners and store in the freezer until you are ready to consume.

This recipe will give you one serving.

Nutritional information per serving:

Calories	150	Carbs	30g	Calcium	22%
Sugar	25g	Protein	8g	Vitamin C	28%
Fiber	2g	Fat	8g		

What You Need:

- Fresh fruit - 1 cup (200g), see below for suggestions
- Non-dairy yogurt - 0.25 cup (50g), see below for suggestions
- Toppings - 0.25 to 0.5 (50g—100g), see below for options

Fruit Suggestions:

- Strawberries, blueberries, raspberries, mango, peaches, bananas.
- Yogurt options:
- Coconut, soy-based or oat milk
- Plain, vanilla, cherry, peach, Pina colada, etc.

*on certain occasions you can switch the yogurt for non-dairy ice cream

Topping Options:

Granola, shredded coconut, cacao nibs, shaved chocolate, sliced almonds, roasted peanuts, etc.

What to Do:

1. In a small bowl, arrange a selection of fresh fruit, scoop a dollop of yogurt on top and sprinkle with an assortment of optional toppings.

This recipe will give you twelve servings.

Nutritional information per serving:

Calories	250	Carbs	34G	Iron	19%
Sugar	20g	Protein	7g	Potassium	4%
Fiber	3g	Fat	18g		

What You Need:

- Non-dairy chocolate chips - 2 cups (400g)
- Peanut butter - 1 cup (200g)
- Coconut oil - 1 tbsp (15ml)
- Vanilla extract - 0.5 tsp (2.5g)

What to Do:

1. In the microwave, melt the coconut oil. Alternatively, you can melt them in a metal bowl over a pot of boiling water.
2. Add the chocolate chips to the melted coconut oil and stir. Once the chocolate is fully melted, with all the chunks gone, stir in the peanut butter and vanilla extract. Stir thoroughly until the peanut butter is evenly distributed.
3. Remove from heat and allow to cool for three to four minutes.
4. Line a shallow, square baking dish with parchment paper. Pour melted chocolate mixture into a lined baking dish, using a spatula to scrape the edges of the bowl.
5. Place the baking dish in the freezer on a flat surface and allow it to cool for three to four hours. Cut into small squares and enjoy two pieces as one serving.

Dessert Ten - Vegan Apple Crisp

You will need twenty minutes to prep and one hour to cook

This recipe will give you ten servings.

Nutritional information per serving:

Calories	310	Carbs	53g	Iron	9%
Sugar	30g	Protein	4g	Vitamin C	14%
Fiber	4g	Fat	12g		

What You Need:

Apple Filling:
- Apples - 8, medium, assorted. four tart (granny smith), four sweet (gala)
- Lemon juice - 1 lemon, squeezed
- Coconut sugar - .75 cup
- Cinnamon - 2 tsp (30g)
- Corn starch - 3 tbsp (45g)
- Apples juice (or water) - 0.25 cup (50ml)
- Grated ginger - 1 tsp (5g) or 0.5 tsp (2/5g) ground ginger
- Nutmeg - 1 pinch

Crumble Topping
- Rolled oats - 1 cup (400g)
- Almond meal - 0.5 cup (100g)
- All-purpose flour - 0.5 cup (100g)
- Coconut sugar - 0.5 cup (100g)
- Brown sugar - 0.5 cup (100g)
- Pecans - 0.5 cup (100g), chopped
- Sea salt - 0.25 tsp (1.5g)
- Cinnamon - 1 tsp (5g)
- Coconut oil - 0.5 cup (100ml), melted

What to Do:

1. Ensure your oven is preheated to 350 degrees Fahrenheit (176 degrees Celsius)
2. Prepare the apples by peeling, coring, and cutting into thin slices, lengthwise.
3. Into a large mixing bowl, add apples, and the rest of the filling ingredients. Toss gently to combine and coat apple slices.

4. Pour apple mixture into a shallow baking dish and distribute in an even layer in the dish.
5. Using the same mixing bowl, prepare the topping. Mix all of the topping ingredients stir.
6. Pour the topping mix over the apples, press topping mix down slightly, but do not pack too tightly.
7. Bake, uncovered, for one hour, or until you see the apple filling bubble up. The topping should be crisp and golden.
8. Remove from the oven, and for thirty minutes, allow it to cool. Serve as-is or with your favorite vanilla non-dairy ice cream.

Dessert Eleven - Healthy Oatmeal Cookies

You will need fifteen minutes to prep and fifteen minutes to cook

This recipe will give you twenty-four servings

Nutritional information per serving:

Calories	75	Carbs	11g	Iron	9%
Sugar	6g	Protein	2g	Calcium	2%
Fiber	1g	Fat	3g		

What You Need:

- Packed dates - 1 cup (200g). Soak for ten minutes in warm water for ten minutes, then drain and pack in measuring cup
- Banana - 1, medium, ripe
- Nut butter - 2 tbsp (30ml). Almond, cashew or peanut butter
- Almond meal - 0.75 cup (150g). Almond meal is more course than almond flour.
- Rolled oats - 0.75 cup (150g)

Optional extras: vegan chocolate chips, dried fruit, seeds, nuts or hemp seed

What to Do:

- In a food processor, add soaked dates and pulse until only small bits remain. Scrap the sides of the processor and ensure all bits are chopped.
- To the food processor, add banana and nut butter. Pulse to combine, scraping the sides as needed.
- Then add the rolled oats and almond meal. Pulse to combine. A crumbly, sticky dough will begin to form.
- Remove the dough from the processor into a medium-sized mixing bowl. Test the dough to see if it forms a ball and stays together. If it doesn't, add a few tbsp of almond meal or oats, or both and stir into the dough until it forms a ball and doesn't stick to your hands.
- Allow the dough to chill in the fridge for ten minutes. If you are using an extra topping, mix into the dough before chilling. 350 degrees Fahrenheit (176 degrees Celsius)
- Onto a medium-sized baking sheet lined with parchment paper, scoop 1 tbsp sized portions of the dough to form a disc. They won't expand but arrange, so the sides are not touching.
- Bake for fifteen to eighteen minutes. They should be golden brown and slightly firm to the touch. It is ok if they are undercooked as there are no eggs to worry about.
- Once golden brown, remove from the oven and let sit for two minutes on the baking sheet, then gently transfer to a cooling rack or plate to continue setting.

Dessert Twelve - No-Bake Chocolate Vegan Brownies

You will need twenty minutes to prep

This recipe will give you twelve servings

Nutritional information per serving:

Calories	390	Carbs	44g	Iron	14%
Sugar	31g	Protein	9g	Magnesium	8%
Fiber	8g	Fat	23g		

What You Need:

Brownie Batter:
- Walnuts - 1.5 cups (150g). 1 cup (100g) for the batter, 0.5 cup (50g) for the topping
- Almonds - 1 cup (100g)
- Dates - 2.5 cups (425g) pitted. Soak in warm water for 10 minutes to soften
- Cacao powder - 0.75 cup (60g)
- Cacao nibs - 2 tbsp (10g)
- Sea salt - 1 pinch

Chocolate Frosting:
- Almond milk - 0.25 cup (60ml)
- Dark chocolate - 1 cup (200g), Egan, chopped
- Coconut oil - 2 tbsp (30ml), melted
- Powdered sugar - 0.25 cup (30g)
- Sea salt - 1 pinch

What to Do:

1. In a food processor, pulse the walnuts and almonds until ground fine
2. Add cacao powder and pinch of salt, pulse again. Scoop mixture out and set aside in a medium-sized bowl.
3. In the food processor, pulse the dates into small bits. Scoop into a separate bowl.
4. In the food processor, add the nut mixture back and pulse. While pulsing add small batches of date pieces through the top of the processor. Pulse until all dates are combined, and you have a dough ball formed in the processor.
5. Line with parchment paper, an 8x8 baking dish. Place half of the dough in the pan, and before pressing, sprinkle in half of the remaining chopped walnuts in roughly even layer. Add the remaining dough and press with your hands into the baking pan. Ensure the dough is firm and flat in the pan.
6. Using the parchment paper, lift the brownies out of the dish. You can lightly squeeze the edges to firm up the sides, making a denser batch of brownies.

7. Place back in the baking dish and place in the fridge or freezer to chill for fifteen minutes while you make the frosting.
8. To prepare the frosting, in a microwave-safe mixing bowl, add the almond milk and warm for forty-five to sixty seconds.
9. Add chocolate to warm almond milk and cover loosely. Allow to rest for two minutes for the chocolate to melt.
10. To the melted chocolate, add a pinch of salt and the melted coconut and stir to incorporate and smooth out any chunks of chocolate that remain. Whisk lightly to distribute the coconut oil thoroughly. Set in the fridge and chill for ten minutes to thicken.
11. Once set, add powdered sugar in small increments, whisking to combine. The frosting will become fluffy.
12. Spread the chocolate frosting over the brownies and sprinkle the last of the chopped walnuts on top.
13. Slice into squares and store in the fridge or freezer.

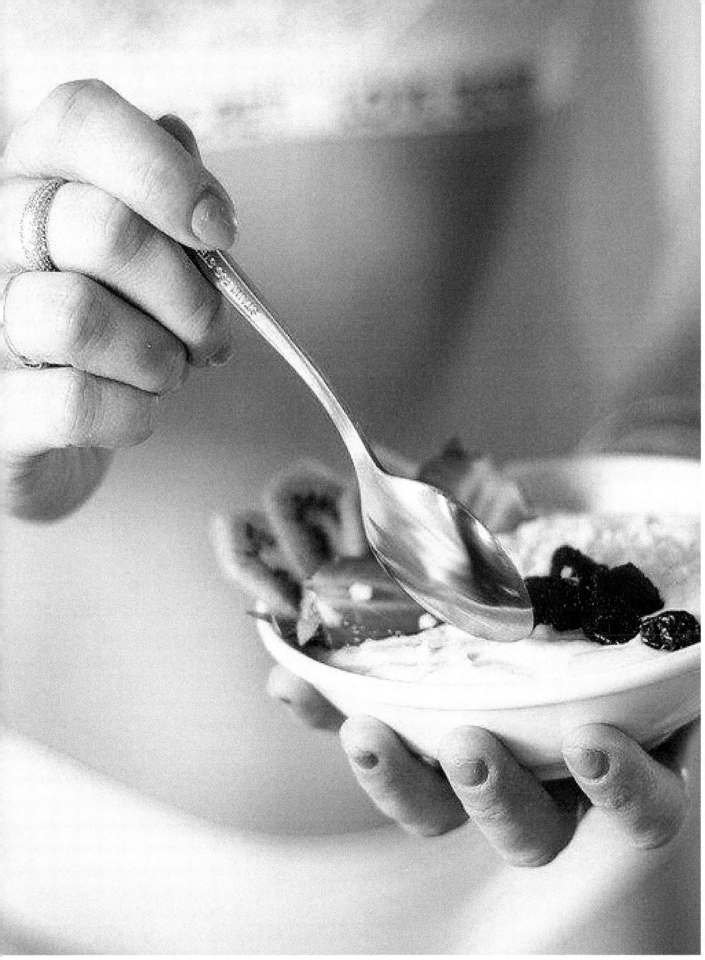

Chapter 11: Recipes for Before & After Workouts

Below are recipes for before and after workouts. These recipes will help you maximize your fitness goals.

Preworkout Recipes

Preworkout: One - Peanut Butter Toast

Nutritional Information Per Serving: 255 Calories, 13 grams of Fat, 26 grams of Carbs, 9 grams of Protein

Time: 5 minutes

Serving Size: 1 serving

Ingredients:
- 1 tablespoon peanut butter
- 1 piece of hearty toast
- ½ banana
- 1 teaspoon chia seeds

Directions:

1. Assemble the toast by toasting the bread, adding the peanut butter, slicing the banana on top, and sprinkling over chia seeds.

Preworkout: Two - Tropical Smoothie

Nutritional Information Per Serving: 455 Calories, 17 grams of Fat, 60 grams of Carbs, 17 grams of Protein

Time: 5 minutes

Serving Size: 1 serving

Ingredients:
- 1 cup frozen mango
- ½ cup pineapple
- 3 cups kale
- 2 tablespoons hemp seeds
- ¼ cup orange juice
- 1 cup coconut milk
- pinch of Himalayan salt

Directions:

1. Add all ingredients into a high-speed blender and blend until smooth.

Preworkout: Three - Apple Slices and Almond Butter

Nutritional Information Per Serving: 162 Calories, 18 grams of Fat, 25 grams of Carbs, 8 grams of Protein

Time: 5 minutes

Serving Size: 1 serving

Ingredients:
- 1 medium apple
- 2 tablespoons almond butter

Directions:

1. Wash and slice the apple before serving alongside almond butter.

Preworkout: Four - Peanut Butter Toast

Nutritional Information Per Serving: 320 Calories, 19 grams of Fat, 25 grams of Carbs, 20 grams of Protein

Time: 5 minutes

Serving Size: 1 serving

Ingredients:
- 8 oz vegan yogurt
- 1 cup blueberries
- ¼ cup almonds, sliced

Directions:

1. Wash the blueberries, and mix all the ingredients together.

Preworkout: Five - Orange and Nuts

Nutritional Information Per Serving: 262 Calories, 21 grams of Fat, 20 grams of Carbs, 4 grams of Protein

Time: 2 minutes

Serving Size: 1 serving

Ingredients:
- 1 orange
- ¼ cup macadamia nuts

Directions:

1. Peel and consume the orange alongside the nuts.

Postworkout Recipes

Postworkout: One - BodyBuilding Smoothie

Nutritional Information Per Serving: 950 Calories, 28 grams of Fat, 154 grams of Carbs, 38 grams of Protein

Time: 5 minutes

Serving Size: 1 serving

Ingredients:
- 2 bananas
- 3 tablespoons chia seeds
- ½ cup chickpeas
- 2 tablespoons dried dates
- 1 tablespoon peanut butter
- 2 cups spinach
- dash of turmeric
- dash of black pepper
- 1 cup soymilk

Directions:

1. Add all ingredients to a high-speed blender and blend until smooth.

Postworkout: Two - Spinach Salad with Tempeh

Nutritional Information Per Serving: 460 Calories, 29 grams of Fat, 29 grams of Carbs, 20 grams of Protein

Time: 15 minutes

Serving Size: 1 serving

Ingredients:

- 3 cups spinach
- 3 oz tempeh, cooked
- ½ cup blueberries
- ¼ cup pecans

Directions:

1. Assemble the salad and add your favorite dressing.

Postworkout: Three - Steel Cut Oats

Nutritional Information Per Serving: 700 Calories, 50 grams of Fat, 64 grams of Carbs, 23 grams of Protein

Time: 5 minutes

Serving Size: 1 serving

Ingredients:
- ½ cup steel oats, dry
- 2 tablespoons peanut butter
- ¼ cup walnuts

Directions:

1. Prepare the oats using the directions on the packaging.
2. Warm peanut butter and pour over the oats when finished.
3. Mix in walnuts.

Note: This can be enjoyed warm or cold. A splash of your favorite plant milk is also welcomed!

Nutritional Information Per Bar: 215 Calories, 15 grams of Fat, 13 grams of Carbs, 11 grams of Protein

Time: 40 minutes

Serving Size: 9 servings

Ingredients:
- ⅓ cup amaranth
- 3 tablespoons vegan protein powder
- 2 tablespoons maple syrup
- 1 cup almond butter
- 3 tablespoons vegan chocolate chips, melted

Directions:

1. Line an 8 x 8 baking pan with parchment paper.
2. Pop amaranth by heating a large pot over medium-high heat. Add amaranth when a drop of water disperses quickly/balls up.
3. Add 2-3 tablespoons amaranth at a time and cover immediately. Shake the pot over the heat to move around the grain. This whole process should take about 10 seconds for the amaranth to pop.
4. Empty the amaranth into a mixing bowl.
5. Add peanut butter and maple syrup into a bowl and stir.
6. Add protein powder. Stir.
7. Add amaranth in small amounts to form a dough.
8. Transfer mixture to baking dish and press down so everything is even.
9. Lay parchment paper over the top and pack the mixture down into a firm, even layer.
10. Place in the freezer for 15 minutes or until firm.
11. Remove pan and slice into about nine bars. Store in the refrigerator until ready to be consumed.

Nutritional Information Per Serving: 540 Calories, 24 grams of Fat, 61 grams of Carbs, 15 grams of Protein

Time: 5 minutes

Serving Size: 1 serving

Ingredients:
- ½ cup hummus of choice
- 5 medium carrot sticks
- 30 multiseed crackers

Directions:

1. Assemble the snack plate by adding hummus, carrots, and healthy crackers.

Conclusion

Over low-calorie pre-packaged snacks, low-carbohydrates homemade meals, and personalized guidance, the Optavia diet encourages weight reduction. When you plan for Optavia to meet the short-term targets of weight reduction, make sure that you are informed about healthier food to hold the weight off during the long term. Further, know that the only method to lose weight is not with a commercial diet where there are restrictions on the calories. Speak to your health professional or a nutritionist about easy adjustments you can take to develop a much more pleasant healthy meal schedule and assist you in meeting your goals. Although the initial 5 and 1 program is somewhat rigid, the maintenance steps of 3 and 3 provide for a wider variety of foods and less refined snacks, making it easier and maintaining weight loss and commitment in the long term. Besides, prolonged restriction of calories can contribute to nutritional deficiencies and other possible health issues.

Whereas the program encourages short-term fat and weight reduction, more study is needed to determine if it encourages the lasting improvements in lifestyle necessary for long-term results. The Optavia Diet may be an excellent choice if you rely on structure and need to shed weight quickly. It's certainly going to help you lose weight with its relatively low-calorie meal plans; though, it's debatable if that weight loss would last once you stop the diet.

Be aware the Optavia goods are not commonly prescribed for any medication or medical problems you have. Often, speaking to individuals who have followed the program, including others who have stopped. An actual view about what the program involves can be given by honest input and suggestions. Before you initiate any nutritional supplement diet carefully evaluate whether you can implement it realistically, assess how much cost you can take, and assess the effect of hunger and disturbance in your daily life and if you are okay with it.

Conversion Charts

VOLUME EQUIVALENTS(DRY)

US STANDARD	METRIC (APPROXIMATE)
1/8 teaspoon	0.5 mL
1/4 teaspoon	1 mL
1/2 teaspoon	2 mL
3/4 teaspoon	4 mL
1 teaspoon	5 mL
1 tablespoon	15 mL
1/4 cup	59 mL
1/2 cup	118 mL
3/4 cup	177 mL
1 cup	235 mL
2 cups	475 mL
3 cups	700 mL
4 cups	1 L

VOLUME EQUIVALENTS(LIQUID)

US STANDARD	US STANDARD (OUNCES)	METRIC (APPROXIMATE)
2 tablespoons	1 fl.oz.	30 mL
1/4 cup	2 fl.oz.	60 mL
1/2 cup	4 fl.oz.	120 mL
1 cup	8 fl.oz.	240 mL
1 1/2 cup	12 fl.oz.	355 mL
2 cups or 1 pint	16 fl.oz.	475 mL
4 cups or 1 quart	32 fl.oz.	1 L
1 gallon	128 fl.oz.	4 L

TEMPERATURES EQUIVALENTS

FAHRENHEIT(F)	CELSIUS(C) (APPROXIMATE)
225 °F	107 °C
250 °F	120 °C
275 °F	135 °C
300 °F	150 °C
325 °F	160 °C
350 °F	180 °C
375 °F	190 °C
400 °F	205 °C
425 °F	220 °C
450 °F	235 °C
475 °F	245 °C
500 °F	260 °C

WEIGHT EQUIVALENTS

US STANDARD	METRIC (APPROXIMATE)
1 ounce	28 g
2 ounces	57 g
5 ounces	142 g
10 ounces	284 g
15 ounces	425 g
16 ounces (1 pound)	455 g
1.5 pounds	680 g
2 pounds	907 g

Lightning Source UK Ltd.
Milton Keynes UK
UKHW050946050121
376451UK00002B/19